Color Atlas of

BREAST DISEASES

Robert E. Mansel, MS FRCS
Professor of Surgery and Head of Department
University of Wales College of Medicine
Cardiff, UK

Nigel J. Bundred, MD FRCS
Senior Lecturer in Surgery
University Department of Surgery
University Hospital of South Manchester
Manchester, UK

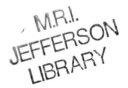

M Mosby-Wolfe

London Baltimore Bogotá Boston Buenos Aires Caracas Carlsbad, CA Chicago Madrid Mexico City Milan Naples, FL
New York Philadelphia St. Louis Sydney Tokyo Toronto Wiesbaden

Copyright © 1995 Times Mirror International Publishers Limited

Published in 1995 by Mosby-Wolfe, an imprint of Times Mirror International Publishers Limited

Printed by Grafos, S.A. Arte sobre papel, Barcelona, Spain

ISBN 0 7234 1721 0

For full details of all Times Mirror International Publishers Limited titles, please write to Times Mirror International Publishers Limited, Lynton House, 7–12 Tavistock Square, London WC1H 9LB, England.

A CIP catalogue record for this book is available from the British Library.

Library of Congress Cataloging-in-Publication Data has been aplied for

Project Manager: Anton Lawrencepulle

Developmental Editor: Claire Hooper

Designer/Layout Artist: Lindy van den Berghe

Cover Design: Lara Last

Illustration: Lee Smith

Production: Jane Tozer

Index: Anita Reid

Publisher: G. Greenwood

Contents

Acknowledgements

Chapter 1: **1.7**, Mr Pye, Wrexham; **1.6** and **1.8**, Dr Tony Douglas-Jones, UWCM, Cardiff; **1.15**, Mr M. Dixon, Edinburgh; **1.19**, Dr Anurag Srivastava, India.

Chapter 5: **5.12**, Dr Anurag Srivastava, India; **5.20** Dr Anurag Srivastava, India.

Chapter 6: **6.8** and **6.9**, Dr V. Naraynsingh, Trinidad, West Indies.

Chapter 7: **7.25**, Mr P. Milewski, Haverfordwest, Wales; **7.26**, Dr Anurag Srivastava, India.

We are grateful to our colleagues in the Surgical Units at University Hospital of Wales (Professor Hughes, Mr Webster, Mr Horgan), Selly Oak Hospital, Birmingham (Mr Morrison), and University Hospital of South Manchester (Professor Sellwood, Mr Baildam, Mr Owen, Dr Asbury, Dr Boggis, Miss Walls) for the use of clinical photographs.

We are also grateful for the help of Professor R. Morton and the Department of Medical Illustration of the University of Wales College of Medicine, and the Medical Illustration Departments of the University Hospital of South Manchester and Selly Oak Hospital.

Preface

It might be considered that an Atlas of Breast Diseases would be a very small volume, as the commonest presentation of breast disease is a lump or nodularity within the breast. However, a surprising number of conditions in the breast do present with clear visible signs representative of a specific condition. The main group is the presentation of cancer in its various forms when it involves the skin, or when it involves other sites by metastasis. Another very large group is the benign conditions which present with inflammation, which are often misinterpreted, but careful study of the enclosed illustrations will give a good guide as to the diagnosis.

Another group of obvious problems which can be diagnosed on sight are many of the nipple disorders, and particularly important is the recognition of Paget's disease, which indicates underlying malignancy.

The imaging of breast conditions is also becoming much more common, and interpretation of mammographic and ultrasound images is now becoming an important part of the work of a specialist breast surgeon.

We hope that this Atlas will enable practitioners to improve their diagnostic ability of common breast conditions without the need for sophisticated technology. We would very much like to acknowledge the help and cooperation of many of our colleagues who have kindly allowed us to use some of their photographs. We hope the reader finds this Atlas enjoyable to read, and educational.

1 Normal Breast

The breasts are identical in both sexes before puberty and are represented by small underdeveloped nipples located on the anterior chest over the fourth intercostal space in the mid-clavicular line. At puberty breast growth commences in the female by elevation of a mound or breast bud beneath the nipple (**1.1**). Breast growth is usually complete by 16–18 years of age.

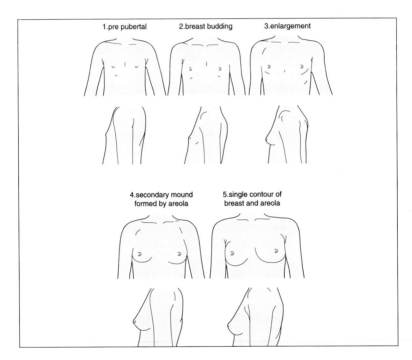

1.1 Breast development. Breast development proceeds in a well-ordered sequence of breast mound elevation, growth and protrusion of the nipple, elevation of a secondary (areolar) mound, and finally regression of the secondary areolar mound to leave the nipple protruding well above the areola.

The adult female breast varies widely in size between individuals and may also vary in an individual when one side is compared with the other. The normal adult breast is roughly conical with a base that extends from the second to the sixth ribs and from the sternal edge to the anterior axillary line (**1.2**). Many developmental anomalies may occur but multiple breast pairs are extremely rare in the human.

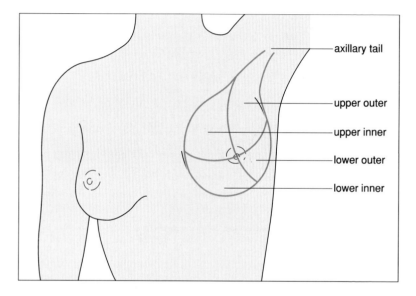

1.2 The normal adult female breast.

Breast activity is mainly related to engorgement and growth in pregnancy in preparing for lactation, although significant cyclical swelling may occur in the luteal phase of the menstrual cycle in many non-pregnant women. The breast doubles in size during pregnancy from an average weight of 200 g to 400 g at delivery. Histologically the resting lobules grow and fill with secretion, so that at term the histological picture is one of large numbers of lobules distended with milk with very little surrounding stroma.

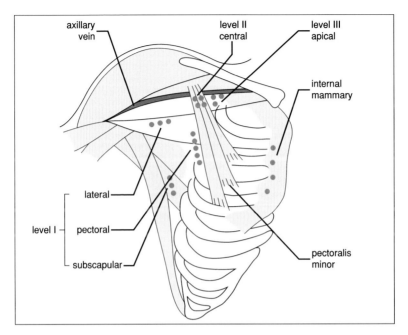

1.3 Axillary lymphatic drainage. Axillary lymph nodes occur at three anatomical levels. Lymph drainage from the breast is via the axillary and internal mammary nodes. To a lesser extent lymph also drains by intercostal routes to nodes adjacent to the vertebrae. The axillary nodes receive approximately 75% of the total lymph drainage and this is reflected in a greater frequency of tumour metastases to these nodes. The axillary nodes which are found below the level of the axillary vein can be divided into three groups in relation to the pectoralis minor muscle: level I nodes lie lateral to pectoralis minor, level II (central) nodes lie behind the pectoralis minor and level III (apical) nodes lie medial to the pectoralis minor muscle between it and the first rib and the axillary vein. There are on average 20 nodes in the axilla with around 13 nodes at Level I, 5 nodes at Level II and 3 nodes at Level III. The drainage from Level I nodes passes into the central nodes and onwards into the apical nodes. There is an alternative route by which lymph can get to Level III nodes without passing through nodes at Level I and that is through lymph nodes on the undersurface of the pectoralis major muscle, the interpectoral nodes.

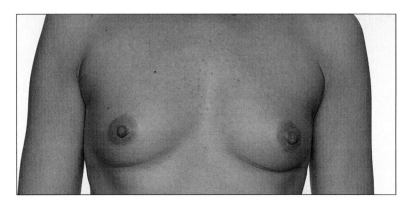

1.4 Normal breasts. In very young women the breasts are symmetrical with pink areolae and normally developed nipples. The breast base is rounded and extends from the second to the sixth ribs and from the sternal edge to the anterior axillary line. The fullness of the pectoralis major muscles is seen above and lateral to the edge of the upper outer quadrant of the breasts.

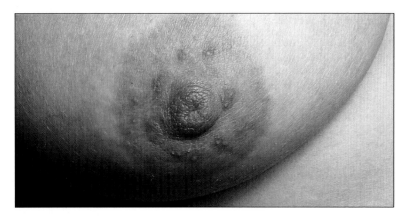

1.5 Normal areola. The skin is slightly pigmented (getting darker in pregnancy) and the surface shows several small irregular nodules which are modified sebaceous glands known as Montgomery's tubercles. The areolar skin and nipple contain a large number of smooth muscle fibres which contract readily to tactile stimulation or exposure to cold.

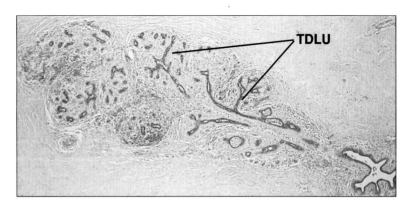

1.6 Normal breast. This longitudinal section through a breast duct arising from a large subareolar duct (in cross section) shows the lobular structure, with several terminal ductal units (TDLU) at the termination of the duct. The loose supporting stroma is well shown. (*H & E stain.*)

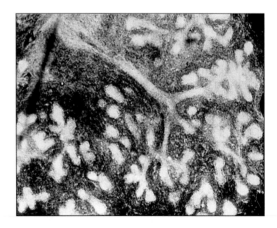

1.7 Microradiograph of normal breast. This is a microradiograph of a 6 micron thick piece of breast tissue taken using the technique of soft tissue microradiography. It shows the elegant multi-branched structure of the breast lobule.

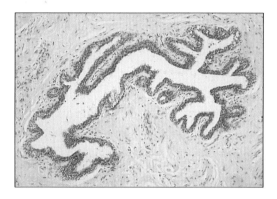

1.8 Transverse section of large subareolar ducts.
The multi-folded appearance of a large subareolar
duct is well shown in this transverse section. The
lax folded wall allows great distension when the
breast is lactating and the duct is full of milk. Note
the simple cuboidal cell epithelium consisting of
two layers of cells. (*H & E stain.*)

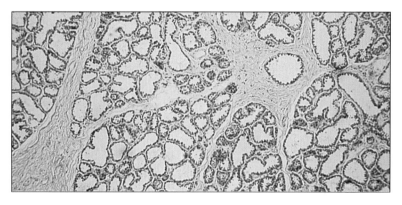

1.9 Lactating breast. Section of lactating breast showing the enormous
distension of the breast alveoli by milk (the empty spaces). The ratio of
epithelium to stroma is much higher than in the resting breast shown in **1.6**.
(*H & E stain.*)

1.10 Enlarged Montgomery's tubercles. The areolar skin shows several enlarged Montgomery's tubercles, the largest one at the areolar margin at 12 o'clock. These changes are due to obstruction of the sebaceous gland duct and can lead to cyst formation or even a superficial abscess if the gland secretions become infected.

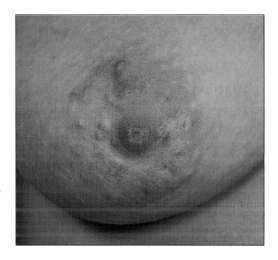

1.11 Supernumerary nipple. An additional nipple or pair of nipples are common and often mistaken for skin warts. This patient has a normally developed nipple and areola (top) and a supernumerary nipple with areola in the lower half of the breast. These additional nipples are usually unconnected with underlying breast tissue as a complete additional breast is much less common. Supernumerary nipples and breasts can occur anywhere along the mammalian milk line extending from axilla to groin.

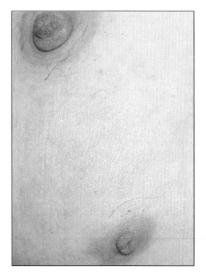

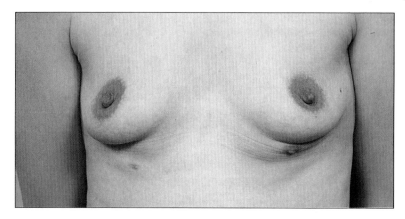

1.12 Supernumerary breast and nipple. This patient shows a complete additional breast on the left side and a supernumerary nipple alone on the right side, both lying below the normal breasts.

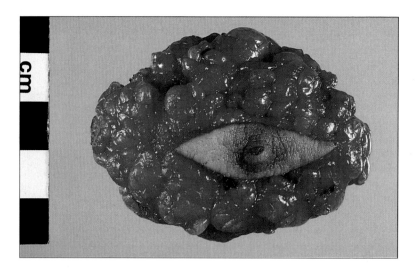

1.13 Excision specimen from the patient in 1.12. This shows a complete breast beneath the nipple and areola. Histological examination revealed normal ducts and lobules separate from the main breast above.

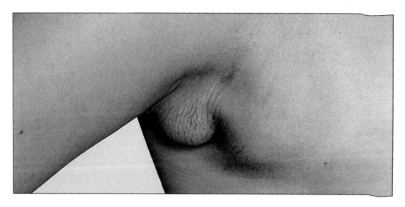

1.14 Accessory axillary breast. Additional breast tissue is often seen in the axilla separate from the breast and may swell cyclically with the menstrual cycle and during pregnancy because it contains normal hormonally-responsive breast tissue. The enlarged axillary mass can be clearly seen in the lower part of this patient's axilla. It proved to be separate from the normal breast on excision, but there was no separate nipple.

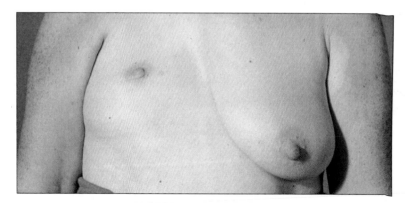

1.15 Poland's syndrome. Abnormal breast development in conjunction with malformation of the underlying pectoral muscle is known as Poland's syndrome. This patient has a malformed right breast with an absent pectoralis major muscle on the right side.

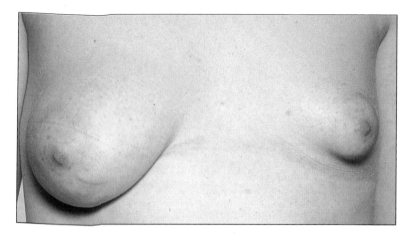

1.16 Breast hypoplasia. Unequal growth of the breasts is common. In this patient the left breast has failed to develop properly although the nipple areola complex is the correct size. This degree of asymmetry requires correction by breast augmentation using an implant.

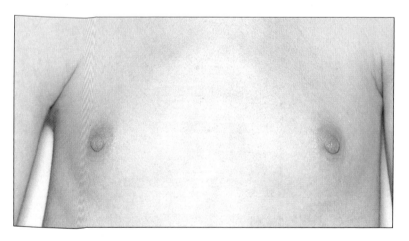

1.17 Total failure of breast development. This 25-year-old patient had radiotherapy to the chest as a child to treat lung metastases from Wilms' tumour. The radiation has totally suppressed normal breast development

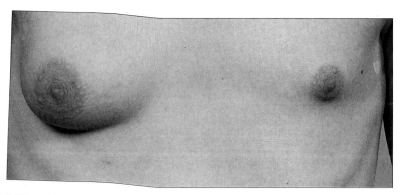

1.20 Pubertal gynaecomastia. This condition is common in boys aged 10–16 years, and may occur in around 30% of normal boys. This 18-year-old man has right-sided gynaecomastia with a definite inframammary fold. The condition usually resolves without treatment, but gross gynaecomastia will require surgical correction. Obese adolescents may appear to have pseudogynaecomastia due to fat. Other causes of gynaecomastia are very rare in pubertal boys.

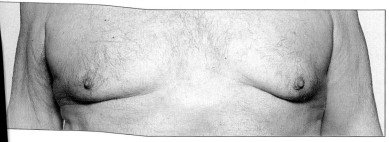

Adult gynaecomastia. This is usually drug-induced (e.g. due to digitalis pironolactone) or secondary to liver disease. This man has moderate eral gynaecomastia due to cimetidine. Secondary gynaecomastia is also in rare conditions such as Kleinfelter's syndrome, testicular tumour, tumour, thyrotoxicosis, and renal failure. It is often seen in body ers when it is caused by the anabolic steroids frequently taken in ng.

1.18 Breast hyper-plasia. This 45-year-old patient has hyper-trophy of both breasts with large pendulous breasts. Such patients suffer pain and find it difficult to wear a bra because the bra straps cut into their should-ers due to the weight of their breasts. Re-duction mammoplasty would be required to correct this.

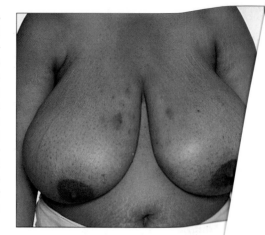

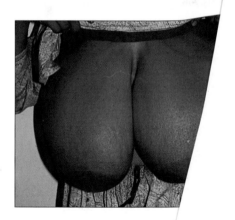

1.19 Virginal hypertrophy. hypertrophy occurs in you uncommon. This patient from and has never been pregn bilateral hypertrophy with which reach her waist. Thi reduction mammoplasty w stopped growing. Some re may help.

1.2
or
bila
seer
lung
buil
train

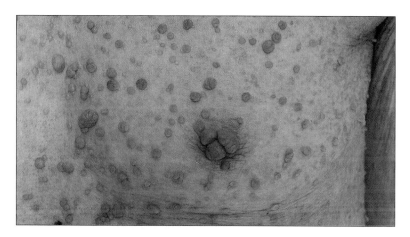

1.22 Neurofibromatosis. People with neurofibromatosis may present with skin lesions over the breast or nipple abnormalities such as the papilloma shown on this nipple. These patients have an increased risk of breast cancer. This patient has already had a right mastectomy for breast cancer.

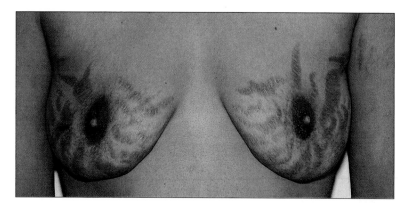

1.23 Adrenogenital insufficiency. Note the marked striae over the breast characteristic of this condition. A similar appearance may occur after pregnancy.

Normal breast examination

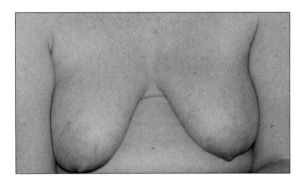

1.24 Normal breast examination: sitting. The patient should be examined in a relaxed sitting position, initially with arms by the side. It is useful to have some light coming from an angle to accentuate any shadows from dimpling of the skin produced by carcinoma. The examiner should look for asymmetry or distortion or altered nipple height.

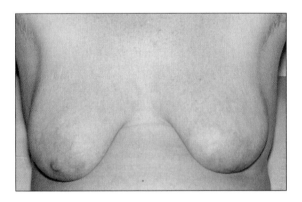

1.25 Normal breast examination: arms raised. The patient should be asked to raise her arms equally in order to look for altered nipple heights or any accentuated dimpling or asymmetry of the breasts.

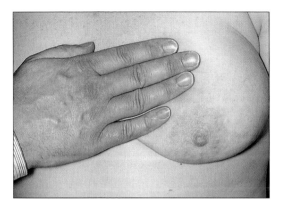

1.26 Normal breast examination: palpating the breast. The breast should be palpated in each quadrant in turn, using the flat of the hand and not the fingertips. The subareolar area should be examined as well as the nipple. The examiner should note any discrete masses and their position within the breast.

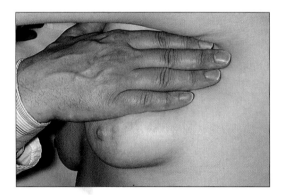

1.27 Normal breast examination: palpation of axilla. The axilla should be examined either from the front or from the back using the fingertips after elevating the arm and bringing it medially in order to relax the pectoralis major muscle. The axillary fat should be rolled against the lateral chest wall in order to detect any nodes which will be felt as lumps between the fingers and rib cage.

2 Worldwide Presentation of Breast Conditions

Breast cancer is the most common form of cancer in women in the USA. Around 183,000 new cases are diagnosed each year in the USA affecting one woman in 10, compared to one in 12 in the UK. The incidence of breast cancer rises steadily with age. Three major risk factors for breast cancer are recognized: age, a family history of breast cancer in a first degree relative, and a history of irradiation at a young age.

Certain countries (e.g. Japan, India) have a low incidence of breast cancer, although Japanese women who move to, or who are born in, the USA develop a fourfold increase in incidence rate. Whether these differences are environmental or genetic is not apparent.

Benign breast disease occurs more commonly in populations at high risk of breast cancer. The majority of women (95%) who present to a breast clinic have benign symptoms and disorders. Diagnosis of breast disorders and disease takes place in the clinic utilising clinical examination, fine needle aspiration cytology and mammography.

The spectrum of benign problems in various countries is similar although black women are more prone to fibroadenoma, whereas Chinese and Caucasian women are more prone to breast cysts.

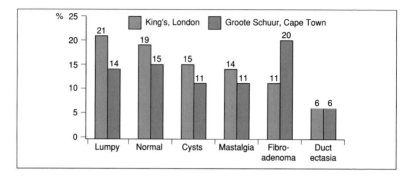

2.1 The prevalence of benign breast complaints is remarkably similar in London and Cape Town. Note that over half of all women presenting to the clinic have variations of normal breast physiology (e.g. nodularity, normal breasts, or mastalgia). There is an increased frequency of fibroadenoma in the South African black population, which is more susceptible to it.

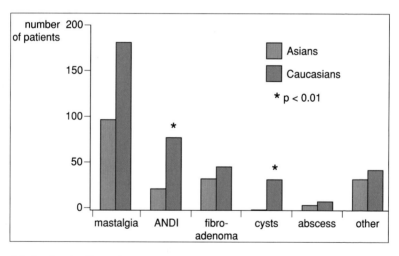

2.2 In the English Midlands, the spectrum of benign disorders is similar. However, Asians are significantly less likely to present with nodular breasts or breast cysts.

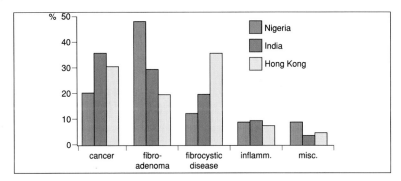

2.3 The Western world has a different pattern of benign breast disease. This is partly because of greater access to medical facilities allowing earlier presentation. In Africa, black populations commonly develop fibroadenoma, but infrequently develop fibrocystic disease or breast cancer. The Hong Kong Chinese however infrequently develop fibroadenoma, but are more prone to breast cysts and breast cancer.

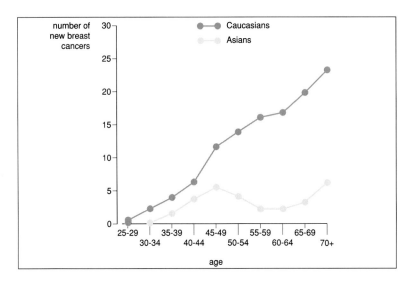

2.4 Breast cancer is much less common in the Asian population in the United Kingdom. Unlike Caucasians, Asian women have a twin peak of breast cancer incidence: the first premenopausal and the second postmenopausal. (Data courtesy of the Trent Cancer Registry.)

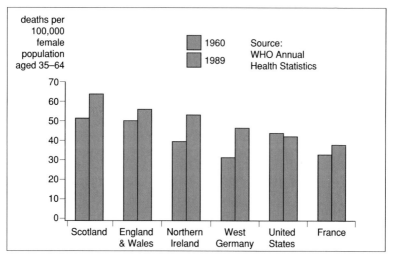

deaths per
100,000
female
population
aged 35–64

1960
1989

Source:
WHO Annual
Health Statistics

70
60
50
40
30
20
10
0

Scotland | England & Wales | Northern Ireland | West Germany | United States | France

2.5 Breast cancer mortality. This is increasing in the United Kingdom and Western Europe, although in the United States deaths from breast cancer are falling. In the United States deaths from heart disease are also declining so the falling breast cancer mortality may reflect changes in diet and lifestyle or the impact of mammographic screening.

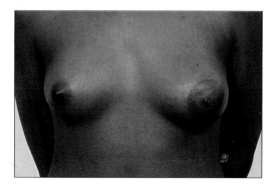

2.6 Giant fibroadenoma. This West Indian girl developed an 8 cm swelling behind the left nipple. This was due to a giant fibroadenoma. Note the enlarged left breast.

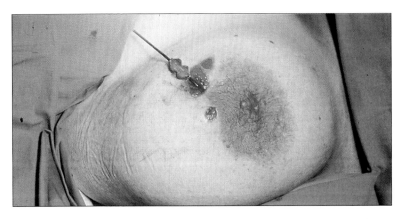

2.7 Mammillary fistulas. These occur in Asian women and are often florid and granulomatous. This woman had two openings into the fistula, which connected with the ducts behind the nipple.

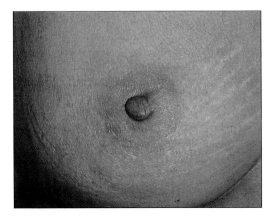

2.8 Breast cancer in Asian women. This lady presented with a swelling behind the right nipple. Note the early nipple retraction laterally.

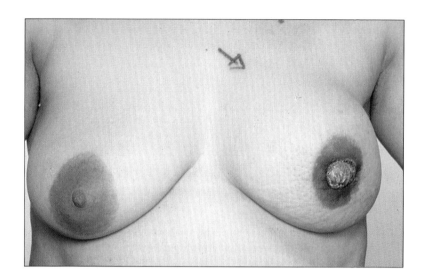

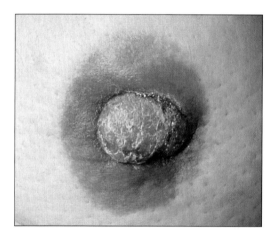

2.9 and 2.10 Nipple infiltration. Infiltration of the nipple may occur with thickening and crusting of the nipple (**2.9**, top). This Asian lady had an advanced breast cancer with peau d'orange of the surrounding breast (**2.10**, bottom).

3 Nipple Disorders and Diseases

Nipple problems are common and can be divided into three main types:

- Nipple inversion.
- Nipple discharge.
- Eczematous conditions.

Nipple Inversion

This ranges from a failure of normal nipple protrusion to frank retraction (**3.2–3.6**). Some form of failure of the nipple to protrude is reported in up to 40% of women and is often noticed only in the teenage years. Such 'congenital' inversion may result from a lack of supporting stromal tissues behind the nipple. The typical transverse nipple retraction presenting in the reproductive years is due to duct ectasia/periductal mastitis, which produces in-drawing due to scarring around the lactiferous ducts contracting and drawing in the nipple. It is often bilateral.

The nipple inversion produced by a subareolar carcinoma is usually very irregular and disordered and is often associated with a palpable mass behind the nipple. The two conditions are easily differentiated radiologically if there is clinical doubt.

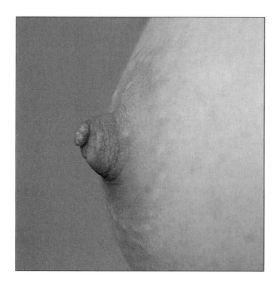

3.1 Nipple papilloma. Nipple papillomas are common and are easily managed by surgical removal.

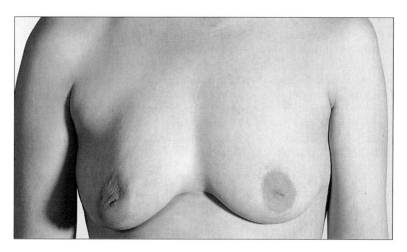

3.2 Congenital nipple retraction. This is present from adolescence and the whole nipple is inverted with no surrounding palpable abnormality. In this girl it is bilateral. Complete retraction makes breast feeding difficult.

3.3 Acquired nipple inversion. The most common cause is periductal mastitis, which produces gradual transverse nipple retraction. This may be unilateral or bilateral.

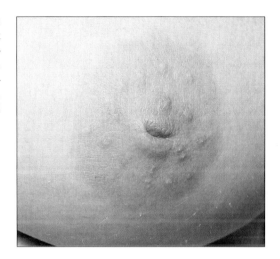

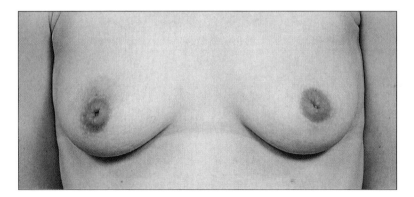

3.4 Periductal mastitis. The nipple retraction of periductal mastitis may be associated with the development of a subareolar mass and inflammation. The condition is associated with heavy cigarette smoking. In this young woman there is bilateral nipple retraction and a mass with visible erythema around the right areola extending into the surrounding breast in the twelve o'clock position.

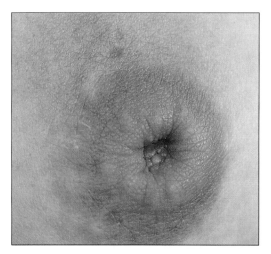

3.5 Periductal mastitis. Close-up view of right breast. The erythema and surrounding oedema are clearly seen and there is obvious nipple retraction.

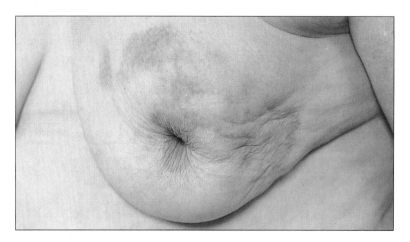

3.6 Nipple retraction due to carcinoma. This patient shows gross irregular nipple retraction due to an underlying carcinoma. Note the additional skin tethering at three o'clock. The bruising is due to previous fine needle aspiration. Nipple retraction of recent onset in postmenopausal women should be investigated by mammography.

Nipple Discharge

Nipple discharge (**3.7–3.13**) comprises 5–10% of all referrals to a breast clinic. It is important when it occurs spontaneously, but if it can be elicited only by squeezing the nipples and breast it is of little consequence. Copious production of breast secretions by manipulating the nipple is common in parous premenopausal women and smokers.

Nipple discharge associated with an underlying lump requires assessment of the mass primarily, but the presence of a mass and a discharge does not increase the likelihood of malignancy. Many women who present with single duct nipple discharge have discharge from multiple ducts that is usually of a coloured nature on examination. Multiple duct discharge is often bilateral, virtually never due to an underlying cancer, and usually caused by duct ectasia. Unless it is copious it is best left alone and the patient reassured. In addition, older women usually require mammography.

The significance of a single duct producing discharge is greater. Frank bloody single duct discharge is normally due to an underlying intraduct papilloma. An underlying nodule will be palpable behind the areola corresponding to the papilloma in about half the patients, or occasionally a thickened duct can be felt. Removal of the underlying duct by microdochectomy will usually reveal a cauliflower-like structure equivalent to the papilloma. Occasionally the bloody discharge will be due to either ductal carcinoma *in situ* or an underlying small carcinoma of the breast. Retroareolar magnification views may help in such diagnosis.

Coloured single duct discharge is usually due to underlying duct ectasia and provided mammography is normal does not require surgery.

3.7 Bloody nipple discharge and lump. The management of associated breast lumps takes precedence over that of a nipple discharge. In this patient the lump was due to an underlying palpable ductal carcinoma *in situ* (shaded area), which produced a profuse bloody discharge from the nipple on compressing the lump.

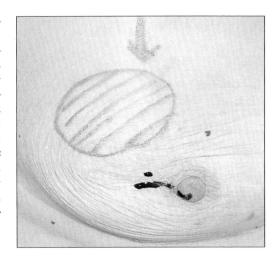

3.8 Multiple duct discharge. This woman presented with nipple discharge that could be expressed from several ducts. It had a dark green colour similar to that of cyst fluid, and this type of discharge is normally benign. Determination of the colour is made easier by examining a drop on a white gauze pad. Although the fluid looks brown on the photograph it appeared dark green on a white gauze. If there is doubt about blood staining this discharge should be tested for blood using a chemical test such as Labstix.

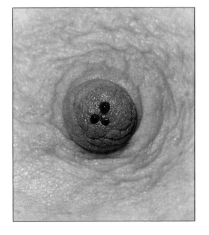

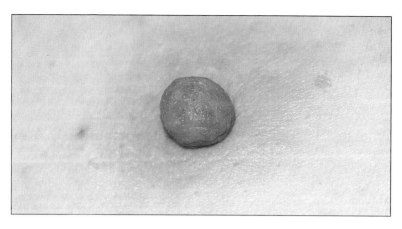

3.9 Single duct discharge. This is more likely to be associated with an underlying malignancy, but overall only about 12% of discharges are associated with malignancy. This patient had a light green single duct discharge which was due to duct ectasia.

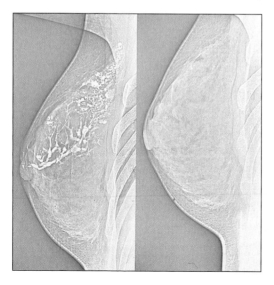

3.10 Ductogram. Injection of contrast medium into the discharging duct showed extensive dilatation of the single duct and its associated branches typical of duct ectasia.

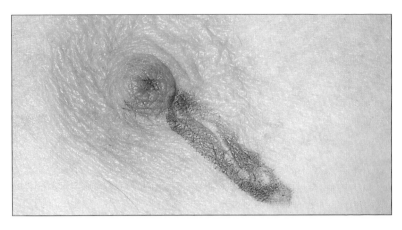

3.11 Bloody single duct discharge. Bloody nipple discharge from a single duct is most often caused by an intraduct papilloma but ductal carcinomas *in situ* need to be excluded. There is often a palpable nodule in the underlying duct which on pressure reproduces the discharge as in this case.

3.12 Intraduct papilloma. The duct is removed at operation and a cauliflower-like projection is commonly found in the duct (arrow). This is a classical benign intraduct papilloma. Serous discharge has the same significance as bloody discharge.

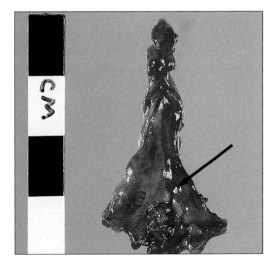

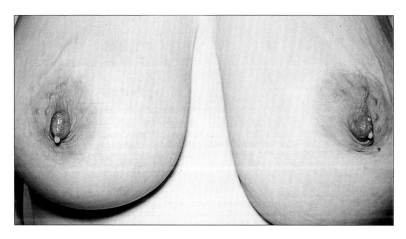

3.13 Galactorrhoea. This patient has milk leaking from both nipples, but she is not pregnant or post-delivery. This is an example of galactorrhoea produced by a prolactin-secreting pituitary tumour.

Eczematous Conditions

Nipple eczema (**3.14, 3.15**) may be entirely localised to the areola and skin, but usually begins on the areola rather than on the nipple and is associated with profuse itching. Generalised nipple areola eczema is rarer and more difficult to distinguish from Paget's disease. If the diagnosis appears to be eczema there is no harm in trying 1% hydrocortisone cream application for a fortnight. Eczema usually responds quickly to hydrocortisone, whereas Paget's disease does not.

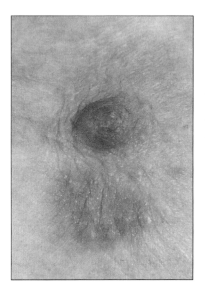

3.14 Early eczema. The inflammation usually begins on the areolar
skin, is associated with itching and
may be the sole manifestation of the
disease. This patient had a hyper-
pigmented papule of eczema at six
o'clock on the areola which
responded to local hydrocortisone
cream.

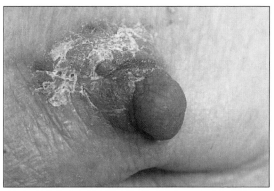

3.15 Scaly eczema. A more florid example with scaling and hyperkeratosis.
Note that in both **3.14** and **3.15** the changes spare the nipple skin and there
is no alteration in nipple anatomy. When there is no erosion of the nipple
surface and no underlying mass, it is reasonable to try a one-month course
of hydrocortisone 1% cream as a diagnostic test as Paget's disease does not
respond to corticosteroids.

Paget's Disease

In contrast to eczema, Paget's disease (**3.16–3.19**) usually begins on the nipple and spreads outwards. It is normally moist (not scaly) and the history is of a continuously evolving lesion that does not respond to corticosteroids. It is always unilateral and the patient complains of itching less often. The nipple is increasingly destroyed.

An elliptical biopsy through the involved skin should be taken under local anaesthetic to confirm a diagnosis of Paget's disease and the patient should always undergo mammography. Rarely there is a palpable underlying mass in women with Paget's disease.

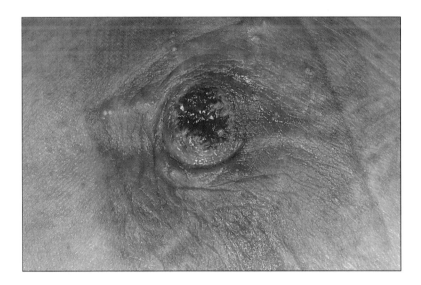

3.16 Early Paget's disease. Paget described this disease in 1874 as an erosion of the nipple with a florid red raw surface. There is usually copious clear discharge from the eroded surface. Microscopically there are large malignant cells with pale cytoplasm and irregular nuclei in clumps in the nipple epidermis. There is usually an underlying breast cancer with a ductal *in situ* component. In the early stages there may be minimal redness of the central nipple skin as shown here.

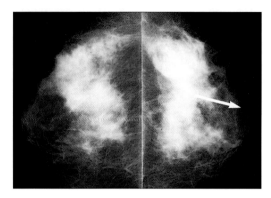

3.17 Mammograms of Paget's disease. These mammograms of the patient in **3.16** show microcalcification in the subareolar ducts behind the left nipple (arrow). Biopsy showed widespread ductal carcinoma *in situ.*

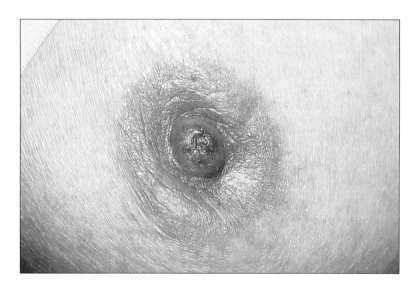

3.18 Pre-erosive Paget's disease. The nipple skin is smooth, reddened, and thickened, although there is no obvious erosion. This is usually due to Paget's disease, but may be due to other conditions such as nipple adenoma (see **3.20**). Biopsy is mandatory to obtain a diagnosis.

3.19 Classic erosive Paget's disease. The nipple is almost completely destroyed and although no underlying mass was palpable, biopsy showed extensive *in situ* cancer requiring mastectomy. If a mass is present it takes precedence in the management.

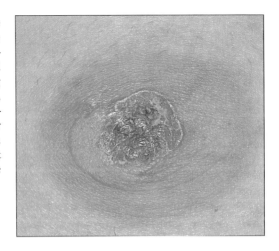

Areolar gland disorders

The areola contains three types of glands within its boundary. Each can cause problems.
• Apocrine sweat glands can become infected or become cystic.
• Sebaceous cysts can occur.
• Occasionally rudimentary mammary glands can develop and give rise to infection or discharge.

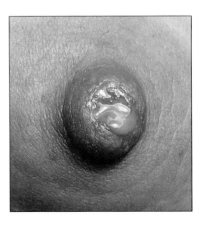

3.20 Nipple adenoma. This is a benign lesion that arises in a nipple duct, but may cause erosion due to pressure necrosis as shown in this example. Wedge biopsy is needed to differentiate it from Paget's disease.

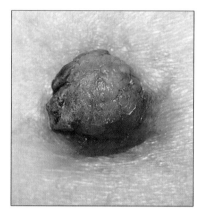

3.21 Lobular carcinoma of the nipple. This is a rare presentation of lobular carcinoma involving the nipple. This postmenopausal lady presented with nipple hardening and no underlying mass: mammography was normal. A wedge biopsy of the nipple under local anaesthetic revealed lobular carcinoma and subsequent mastectomy failed to reveal any other malignant change in the breast. Note the changes are confined to the nipple.

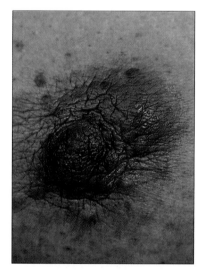

3.22 Areolar cysts. An example of an areolar cyst at two o'clock arising from an apocrine gland in the areolar skin. This had become infected and required excision.

4 Mastalgia

Mastalgia (breast pain) is one of the commonest reasons for consultations for breast problems. Studies have shown that up to 60% of women experience some degree of mastalgia at some time and the symptom is the predominant reason for referral in 40% of women who attend the breast clinic. After investigation and reassurance of the absence of cancer, only some 20% of referred patients require drug treatment. As with any of the common presenting symptoms of breast disease a careful clinical examination is needed to exclude breast lumps suspicious of carcinoma. Generalised nodularity is common in mastalgia, especially in the cyclical subgroup. Treatment is indicated for patients who suffer at least seven days of severe pain each month and can be monitored by using a pain chart.

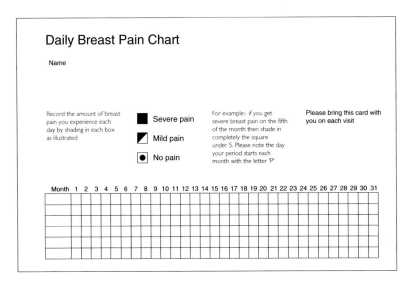

4.1 Standard Cardiff pain chart. This chart is used to estimate the qualitative and quantitative effects of breast pain. The patient records pain severity each day of the cycle and records the onset of menstruation (if still menstruating).

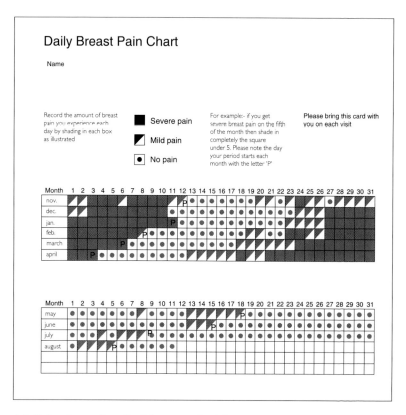

4.2 Pain chart of cyclical breast pain. This chart shows a typical cyclical pronounced pattern of pain for more than seven days per cycle, mostly occurring in the luteal or pre-menstrual phase of the cycle. This pattern is the most common and occurs in 66% of women with mastalgia, with a varying duration of pain from seven days to almost the whole cycle. Nodularity is common and the pain is described as 'heaviness' or 'tenderness to touch'. The lower panel shows the pain chart of the same patient on successful therapy indicating that it is an excellent method of measuring the response to therapy.

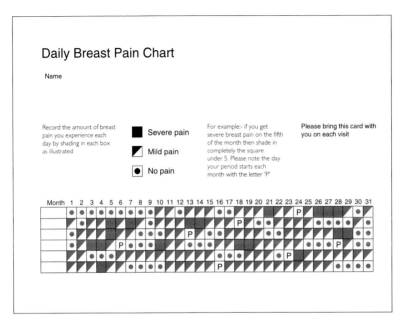

Daily Breast Pain Chart

Name

Record the amount of breast
pain you experience each
day by shading in each box
as illustrated

■ Severe pain

◢ Mild pain

● No pain

For example:- if you get
severe breast pain on the fifth
of the month then shade in
completely the square
under 5. Please note the day
your period starts each
month with the letter 'P'

Please bring this card with
you on each visit

4.3 Pain chart of non-cyclical breast pain. A pain chart showing a pattern of pain unrelated to the menstrual cycle. This type of mastalgia occurs in both pre- and postmenopausal women. In non-cyclical pain causes outside the breast such as pain from cervical spondylosis or Tietze's disease should be considered. The pain is often described as 'drawing' or 'burning' and nodularity is uncommon.

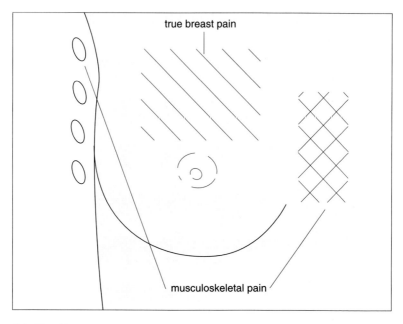

true breast pain

musculoskeletal pain

4.4 Classification of non-cyclical breast pain. Non-cyclical pain can be divided into true breast pain arising from the breast tissue or musculoskeletal pain arising from the ribs or chest wall. Musculoskeletal pain is common medially (Tietze's syndrome) or laterally at the edge of the breast. Examining the patient while leaning forward to make the breast fall away from the chest wall allows better differentiation of these subtypes.

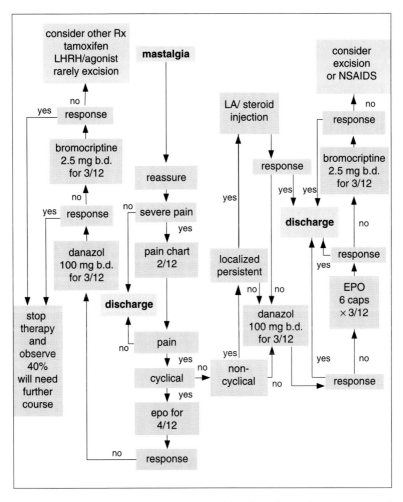

4.5 Flow chart of mastalgia treatment. The flow chart gives a suggested management protocol for those patients requiring treatment for their mastalgia. Adequate reassurance should always be given before treatment is started as this will be sufficient for some 80% of women with mild or moderate mastalgia. (EPO, evening primrose oil; NSAIDs, nonsteroidal anti-inflammatory drugs.)

5 Inflammation and Infection in the Breast

Breast inflammatory conditions are uncommon and often inappropriately managed. Under 6% of all breast surgery is performed for breast inflammation, but in some series up to one third of patients suffer recurrent symptoms or postoperative complications.

The clinical syndrome of periductal mastitis is responsible for the majority of patients with breast inflammation and infection seen in the UK and USA. Periductal mastitis is characterised by subareolar inflammation associated with the development of recurrent nonlactating breast abscesses, mammillary fistulae, transverse nipple retraction or coloured nipple discharge. Anaerobic and aerobic bacteria are often found associated with the lesions of periductal mastitis, and cigarette smoking has recently been implicated as a cause of the disease.

It is important to use antibiotics to treat the early stages of the disease and as prophylaxis for any surgical operations.

Other inflammatory conditions of the breast (e.g. fat necrosis, tuberculosis) occur but are rare manifestations. Tuberculosis tends to be more common in Asian and black women. Mondor's disease (superficial thrombophlebitis of veins on the breast) occurs either spontaneously or after a surgical incision. The thrombosed vein is usually visible and can be palpated by rolling it underneath the finger when it is felt as a cord within the breast.

Breast Abscess

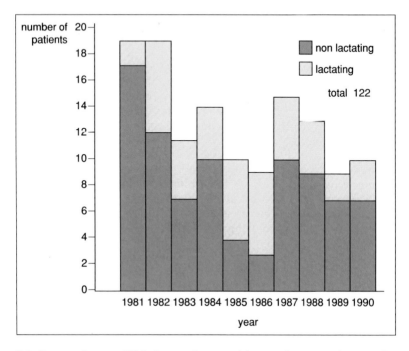

5.1 Breast abscess. With improving nutrition and postnatal care, the frequency of lactational breast abscess is declining. Lactational abscesses are nearly always associated with *Staphylococcus aureus* infection in contrast to non-lactational breast abscesses, which are associated with a mixture of organisms including coliforms and anaerobes. The incidence of non-lactational abscesses, which are usually subareolar in site, is increasing so that in hospital practice they account for two of every three breast abscesses seen.

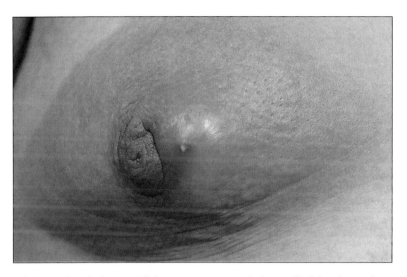

5.2 Lactational abscess. This may present early in a cellulitic phase when treatment with antibiotics may lead to resolution or at a phase when pus is aspirated from the breast and surgical intervention is usually required. This patient had extensive nipple oedema due to the underlying abscess and could not continue breastfeeding, but usually expression of the breast milk will help to reduce congestion and resolution. Flucloxacillin is the antibiotic of choice for this predominantly staphylococcal infection. Note that the abscess is 'pointing' at three o'clock on the areolar margin and will need surgical drainage for treatment.

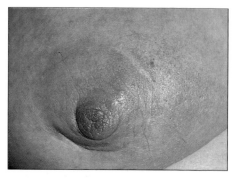

5.3 Non-lactational breast abscesses. These occur in women in their mid-30's and indicate underlying periductal mastitis. They are common in cigarette smokers and tend to recur. Acute abscesses can be treated by aspiration of pus and antibiotic therapy. The presence of non-staphylococcal organisms in a non-lactational breast abscess should alert the clinician to the possibility of underlying duct ectasia or a mammary fistula. Most commonly coliform or anaerobic bacteria are present in the pus and antibiotics directed at such organisms are necessary (e.g. co-amoxiclav or metronidazole). Note the old circumareolar scar at one o'clock indicating a previous episode of periductal infection requiring surgery.

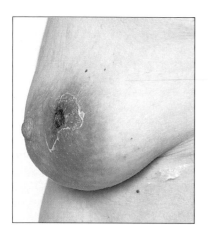

5.4 Chronic non-lactational abscess. A long-standing abscess showing overlying skin necrosis. It had discharged spontaneously. Such spontaneous discharge commonly leads to an established mammary duct fistula. At this stage surgery is always required to drain the abscess properly.

Periductal Mastitis

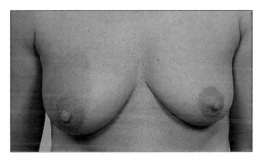

5.5 Early periductal mastitis. The inflammatory phase before abscess formation. Clinically there is a flame-shaped tender erythematous area forming outwards from the areola at twelve o'clock in the right breast. This corresponds to the underlying histological picture of periductal cuffing with acute inflammatory cells without duct dilatation. There is marked induration with oedema, but no pus formation.

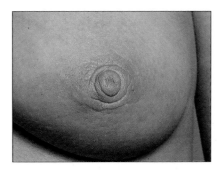

5.6 Early periductal mastitis with oedema. The marked oedema has caused peau d'orange of the lower areola and breast skin. Note the marked nipple oedema. The appearance may mimic inflammatory carcinoma, but that condition is usually painless. Treatment is with antibiotics with review in one week. If there is no resolution, further diagnostic investigations are indicated.

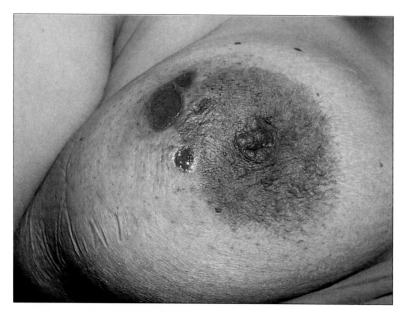

5.7 Mammillary fistula. Spontaneous discharge may occur following acute periductal mastitis, classically at the areolar edge, and lead to an established mammillary fistula. This patient has two external openings at nine and ten o'clock on the areolar edge of her right breast.

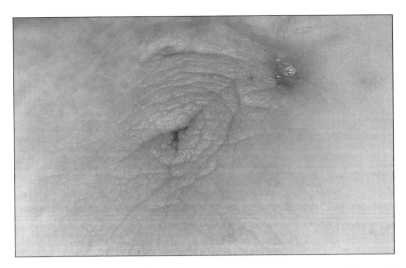

5.8 Mammillary fistula after abscess drainage. After simple incision and drainage of a non-lactational abscess there is a high risk of a fistula developing along the scar tract from the skin to the underlying ducts. This patient demonstrates a classic fistula at the lateral edge of her drainage scar. Note the transverse retraction of the nipple typical of long-standing duct ectasia.

5.9 Chronic mammary duct fistulae. This patent has undergone at least twelve operations in an attempt to cure mammary duct fistulae. Note the extensive scar and cavity with the fistula opening at the base. Cure of these fistulae requires careful subareolar dissection with accurate identification and excision of the involved ducts under antibiotic cover. Primary closure without antibiotic cover leads to a 30% rate of recurrence.

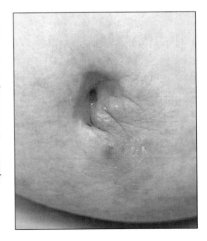

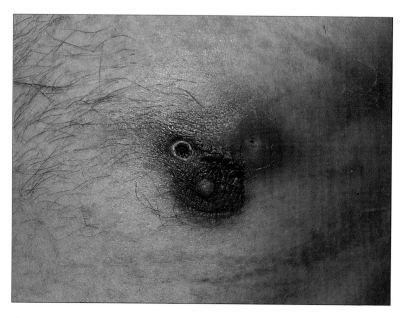

5.10 Male mammary duct fistula. This ductal disease can occur in males because they have major lactiferous ducts. This man smoked 40 cigarettes a day (an important factor in periductal fistula formation in women) and developed an abscess with subsequent fistula formation. He also had human immunodeficiency virus (HIV) infection.

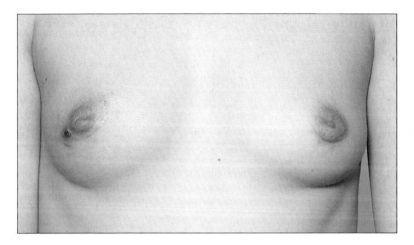

5.11 Bilateral periductal mastitis. Periductal mastitis occurs in a wide age range, but subareolar sepsis (abscess and fistula) predominates in young women. This 15-year-old girl developed bilateral subareolar sepsis and was also a cigarette smoker. Note the erythema of both sides with a fistula of the right breast.

5.12 Postoperative milk fistula. Biopsy of the lactating breast carries the hazard of a subsequent milk fistula. This patient had a biopsy for a hard nodule, but subsequently developed a milk fistula. Note the milk coming from the nipple and the wound on compressing the breast. Fine needle aspiration cytology should be the preferred diagnostic method in lactating women.

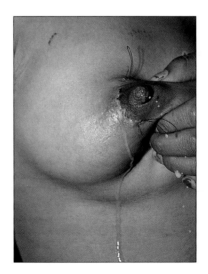

Mammillary Fistulae: Management

Mammillary fistulae (**5.13–5.18**) are abnormal communications between lactiferous ducts and the breast skin. Treatment of this condition can be difficult and various methods suggested include laying open the fistula, excision and primary closure with or without antibiotic cover, excision and secondary closure without antibiotic cover, and total duct excision. Usually not just the duct associated with the fistula, but all the ducts of the breast are affected by periductal mastitis, and the treatment of choice is a fistulectomy combined with a total duct excision through a circumareolar incision.

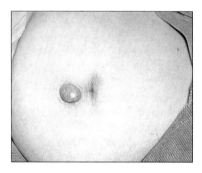 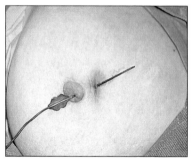

5.13 Mammillary Fistulae. Nipple discharge occurs from the affected duct on pressure over the fistula. This woman smoked 40 cigarettes a day and had a breast abscess which discharged itself spontaneously producing a fistula. Mammillary fistulae may also present after surgical biopsy of the breast or after incision and drainage of a subareolar abscess in a nonlactating breast.

5.14 A probe passed through the discharging duct emerges from the fistula opening.

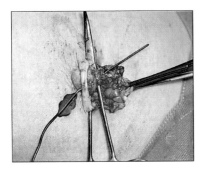

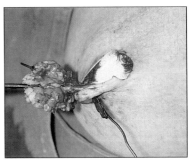

5.15 Using a circumareolar incision including the existing fistula opening, the fistula and major ducts are dissected free.

5.16 The specimen is elevated before division of all the ducts at the base of the nipple.

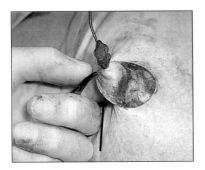

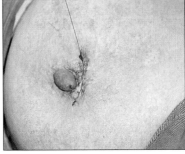

5.17 The nipple's inverted base is showed free of all major ducts and a purse-string suture may be used to evert the nipple.

5.18 Primary closure is carried out with a subcuticular suture under antibiotic cover.

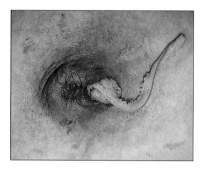

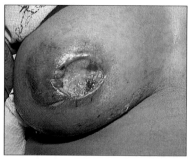

5.19 Fistulectomy and packing. If primary closure is difficult due to a large chronic subareolar abscess cavity an alternative management technique is to excise the fistula and pack the cavity.

5.20 Packing after fistula excision. This patient is shown after treatment of a large abscess with subsequent packing. The wound is an ideal shape with a flat saucer-shape cavity, which will heal readily by granulation. The final scar may be quite good after this procedure.

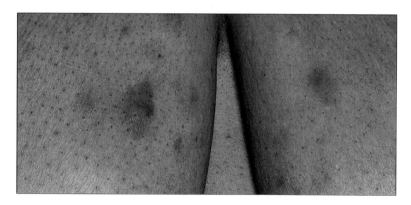

5.21 Infected sebaceous cyst. Occasionally a sebaceous cyst of the breast skin becomes infected and requires antibiotic treatment with or without drainage before excision. It is important not to confuse such a lesion with hidradenitis suppurativa of the breast. The sebaceous cyst is seen in the upper half of the right breast.

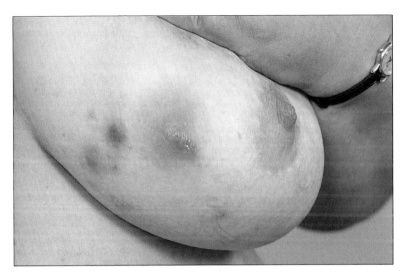

5.22 Hidradenitis suppurativa. This is a disease of the apocrine sweat glands found mainly in the axilla and groins, but also in the inframammary folds and areola. Disease on the breast may occur without any other involved sites. The treatment is skin excision and packing, allowing healing by secondary granulation. The lesions are multiple and often widely spaced as shown in this patient.

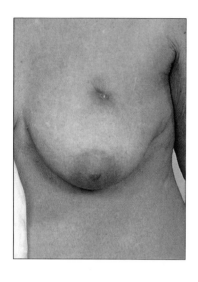

5.23 Primary tuberculosis of the breast. Tuberculosis of the breast is rare and in the UK tends to occur in the immigrant population. In India it remains common. It may present as sinuses, ulcers, a contracted breast, or a cold abscess. A deltopectoral (infraclavicular) cold abscess is not uncommon. Antituberculosis chemotherapy may not completely eradicate the disease and mastectomy is required. This Pakistani patient presented with a deep sinus in the breast, which histologically showed typical granulomatous inflammation. The inflammation originated in the breast tissue and there was no evidence of pulmonary tuberculosis.

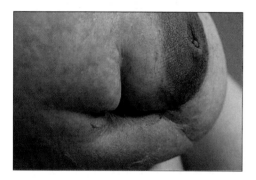

5.24 Secondary breast tuberculosis. This woman presented with a grossly deformed contracted breast and multiple sinuses in the fissures seen on the skin. On surgical exploration these communicated with similar inflammation in the pleural space. The breast was therefore secondarily involved by tuberculosis originating in the pleural space.

5.25 Breast tuberculosis: mammogram. This mammogram shows extensive inflammation in the breast of the patient seen in **5.24**. The track leading to the pleural space can be seen extending posteriorly upwards from the lower half of the breast (arrow).

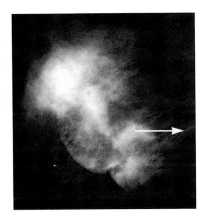

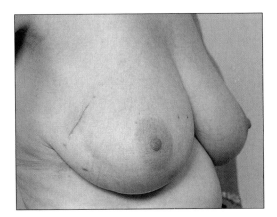

5.26 Postoperative Mondor's disease. The patient noted a groove in the skin following a recent breast biopsy and this is seen in the right breast below the scar. Mondor's disease settles spontaneously and non-steroidal anti-inflammatory drugs are useful for pain relief.

5.27 Spontaneous Mondor's disease. This more common presentation is probably caused by minor trauma. The thrombosed vein in the subcutaneous tissue below the left breast is seen as a raised cord.

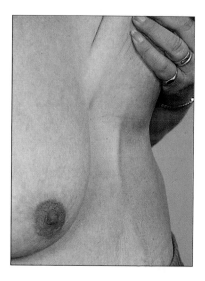

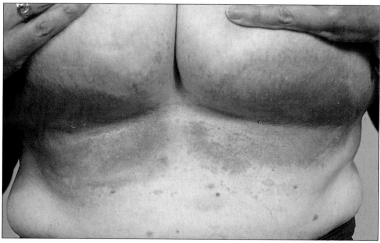

5.28 Inframammary fold intertrigo. Classic inframammary infection typically seen in older women with large pendulous breasts. This is due to fungal infection such as *Candida*.

6 Breast Lumps

Dominant breast lumps occur in three distinctive age ranges in women. Among those aged 12–35, fibroadenoma is the commonest lump; in women aged 35–55 breast cysts are common, and in women above 55, most lumps are due to cancer (**6.1**).

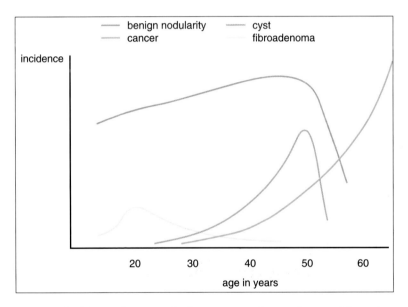

6.1 The incidence by age of the common breast lumps. Note that fibroadenoma occurs in the young woman and cysts in the perimenopausal woman. Cancer begins at about 25 but is only common from the age of 45 onwards. Benign nodularity is common in young women and persists until the menopause at 50; this condition is often mistaken for a discrete lump by women.

There is a considerable overlap in the age range between cysts and carcinoma, especially in the 40–55 age group when the incidence of cancer is rapidly rising. Other causes of lumps such as inflammatory conditions of the breast are seen in all age groups. It is important to differentiate between a dominant lump and areas of nodularity, which can occur at any age, although much more commonly between the ages of 20–50 years. Dominant lumps have discrete borders and are usually measurable with callipers. The surface consistency is important as the smooth rounded surface of a cyst contrasts markedly with the hard irregular surface of a cancer. The most difficult masses are those with an area of increased hardness within an existing area of nodularity although imaging by mammography and ultrasound will usually determine whether a discrete mass is present or not.

ANDI

Most benign lesions can be described within the new ANDI (Aberrations of Normal Developmental and Involution) classification, which describes these lesions as benign breast conditions rather than diseases (**6.2**). This is a more appropriate classification as it correctly suggests that most benign lesions are changes from the normal physiological state and carry no increased risk of breast cancer.

ABERRATIONS OF NORMAL DEVELOPMENT AND INVOLUTION (ANDI)

STAGE	NORMAL PROCESS	ABERRATION		DISEASE STATE
		Underlying Condition	**Clinical Presentation**	
EARLY REPRODUCTIVE LIFE (15–25)	Lobule formation	Fibroadenoma	Discrete lump	Giant fibroadenoma Multiple fibroadenoma Phylloides tumour
	Stroma formation	Juvenile hypertrophy	Excessive breast development	
MATURE REPRODUCTIVE LIFE (25–40)	Cyclical hormonal effects on glandular tissue and stroma	Exaggerated cyclical effects	Cyclical mastalgia and nodularity generalised or discrete	
INVOLUTION (35–52)	Lobular involution (including micro-cysts, apocrine change, fibrosis adenosis)	Macrocysts sclerosing lesions	Discrete lumps X-ray abnormalities	
	Ductal involution (including periductal round cell infiltration)	Ductal dilatation Periductal fibrosis	Nipple discharge Nipple retraction	Periductal mastitis with bacterial infection and abscess formation
	Epithelial turnover	Mild epithelial hyperplasia	Histological report	Epithelial hyperplasia with atypia

6.2 Aberrations of Normal Development and Involution (ANDI) classification.

Fibroadenoma

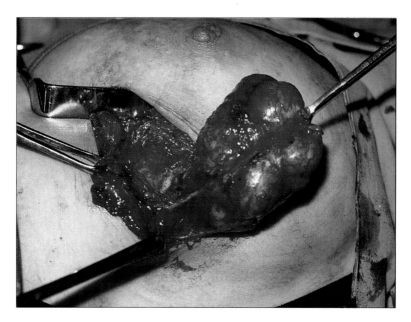

6.3 Fibroadenoma. Operative photograph of excision of a typical multilobulated fibroadenoma. These present in young women as solitary mobile discrete lumps (breast mouse). They are solid on aspiration and have a characteristic appearance on ultrasound. In women less than 35 years of age they may be left *in situ* provided both the cytology and ultrasound are benign. In women over 35 years of age they are usually removed.

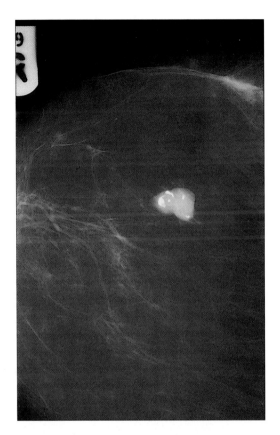

6.4 Mammogram of fibroadenoma. Note the discrete well-defined margins and homogeneous density with typical benign calcification within the lesion. These lesions are frequently seen on screening mammography and are usually left because they are asymptomatic and benign. If there is any doubt about their nature cytology is performed.

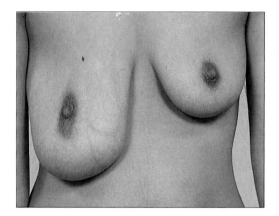

6.5 Giant fibroadenoma. Large fibroadenomas often distend the breast by their bulk as in this patient with a grossly enlarged right breast. The mass was clearly well-demonstrated, mobile, and rubbery in texture. The patient complained of pain in the right breast around the lump.

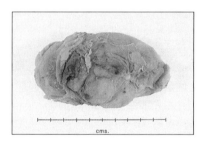

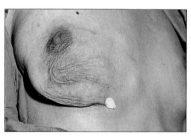

6.6 Operative specimen of giant fibroadenoma. The lesion measured 10 cm in diameter and showed evidence of infarction, which explained the pain that the patient had noticed.

6.7 Immediate postoperative result. An inframammary approach (Gaillard) was used to remove the mass. Note the lax skin and breast tissue after removal of the large mass. The breast gradually returns to a normal shape.

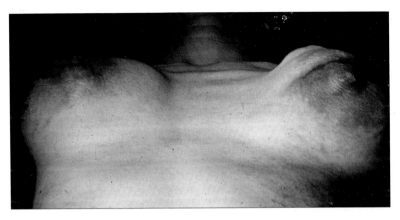

6.8 Familial fibroadenomas. Rarely there is a familial tendency for fibroadenoma formation, usually in Asian races. This patient from the West Indies presented with large numbers of fibroadenomas as did her daughter.

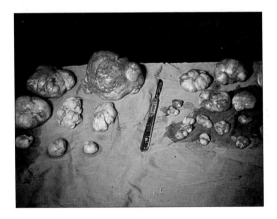

6.9 Familial fibroadenomas. The surgical excision specimen shows eight fibroadenomas removed from one side and sixteen from the other. (The scalpel lies between the two groups of fibroadenomas.)

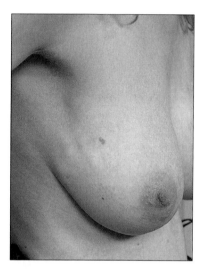

6.10 and 6.11 Cyclosporin-induced fibroadenoma. A rare presentation of multiple fibroadenomas induced by cyclosporin A. This patient had had a renal transplant and developed multiple fibroadenomas, which can be seen indenting the breast skin (**6.10**, upper). These grew rapidly, but appeared as typical fibroadenomas on ultrasound (**6.11**, lower). Compared with the ultrasound appearance of a cyst (see **6.15**), the lesion is well-defined, but solid.

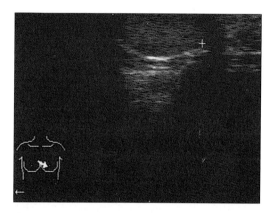

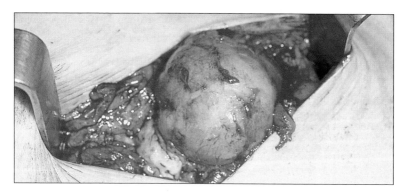

6.12 Cystosarcoma phylloides. This tumour is generally benign, but often recurs locally if inadequately examined. It presents as a discrete growing mass that is clinically indistinguishable from a large fibroadenoma. About 10% are found to be malignant from the outset, but these are usually fast growing and recur rapidly following excision. Recurrence after an adequate excision suggests that mastectomy is needed.

Cyst

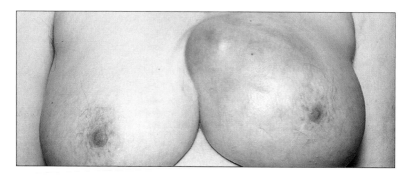

6.13 Breast cyst. This is an unusually large cyst. Most are palpable rather than visible. About 7% of women in the Western world are said to develop breast cysts.

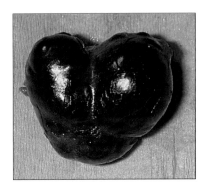

6.14 Blue-domed cyst of Bloodgood. This excised cyst appears blue due to the pigmented nature of the contained fluid. Such cysts are usually treated by simple aspiration when easily palpable.

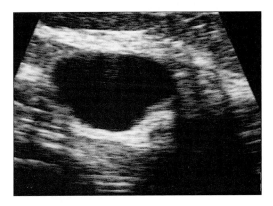

6.15 Ultrasound of breast cyst. The ultrasound appearance is characteristic with a clear rounded lesion and no internal echoes or acoustic shadowing. Most palpable cysts can be aspirated without radiological imaging, but deep-seated or screen-detected lesions may be better defined with ultrasound.

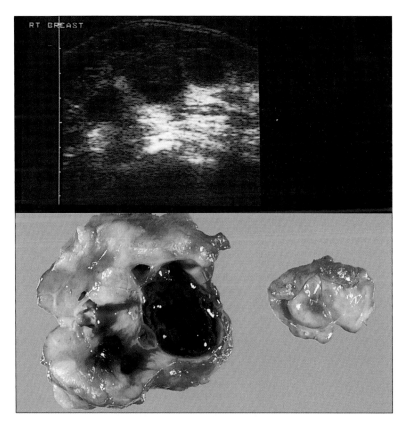

6.16 Ultrasound and operative specimen. Cysts are commonly multiple and 50% of women who have a cyst aspirated will go on to have further cysts. This patient had an aspiration with rapid refilling of the cyst and the ultrasound showed a solid area in the middle cyst shown by the internal echoes. At operation, this proved to be due to a haematoma following the aspiration.

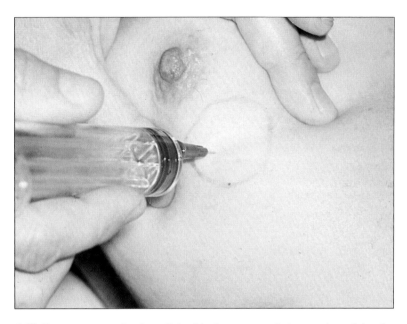

6.17 Breast cyst aspiration. Palpable breast cyst being aspirated in the outpatient clinic. The cyst is steadied between the finger and thumb of the left hand and the needle is passed into the centre of the cyst. On entering the cyst fluid appears in the barrel of the syringe and a characteristic 'give' is felt. The cyst should be aspirated to dryness. If there is blood in the cyst fluid or the lump is still palpable after aspiration then cytology and mammography are indicated as a carcinoma may be present. Cytology of non-blood stained cyst fluid is unnecessary.

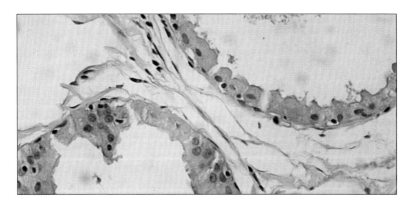

6.18 H & E section of breast cysts. Cells lining breast cysts are either flattened or more commonly have apocrine characteristics. This section shows classic apocrine epithelium consisting of tall columnar eosinophilic cells, with basally situated nuclei and apical snouts.

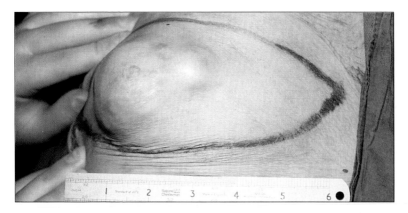

6.19 Intracystic carcinoma. Rarely, breast cysts occur for the first time in elderly women taking hormone replacement therapy. Intracystic carcinoma should always be suspected if a new cyst appears in a previously asymptomatic elderly patient and cytology should be obtained. Cytology of this patient's cyst proved to be malignant and she was admitted for mastectomy.

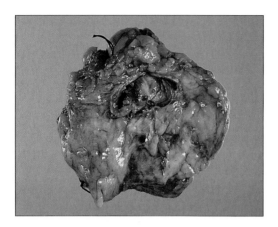

6.20 Intracystic papilloma. If after cyst aspiration the lump fails to disappear the residual mass should be excised. In this case the cyst contained a benign intracystic papilloma. The papilloma is seen in the centre of the cyst after excision.

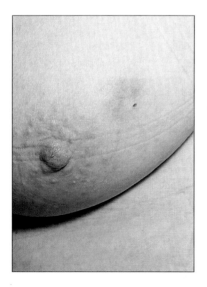

6.21 Sebaceous cyst. Any skin lesion may occur on the breast skin. This patient presented with a classic sebaceous cyst seen at two o'clock outside the areolar margin. Note the classic punctum with firm sebaceous plug (blackhead).

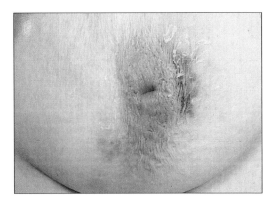

6.22 Fat necrosis. This presents as a hard mass in the breast following an episode of trauma sufficient to cause bruising. This patient shows bruising secondary to a deceleration injury caused by a seat belt and an underlying mass was present. The mass remained for at least one month after the bruising had disappeared. The diagnosis should be confirmed by cytology, mammography, and ultrasound. Occasionally trauma may draw the patient's attention to a pre-existing carcinoma.

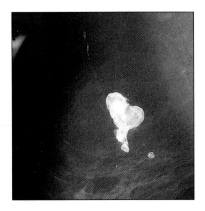

6.23 Mammogram of fat necrosis. Long-standing fat necrosis may calcify as shown on this mammogram.

7 Breast Cancer: Presentation

About 80% of symptomatic breast carcinoma presents as a palpable mass. Less common presentations are nipple discharge and retraction, Paget's disease, or an axillary mass. Advanced presentations include skin ulceration, skin nodules, and the skin oedema known as peau d'orange. Increasingly, impalpable cancers are detected by screening mammography and have no clinical signs. Examination of a patient with a suspected breast cancer follows the usual inspection and palpation technique. Diagnostic investigations will include mammography, ultrasound, and tissue diagnosis by fine needle aspiration cytology or thick needle core biopsy (Trucut™).

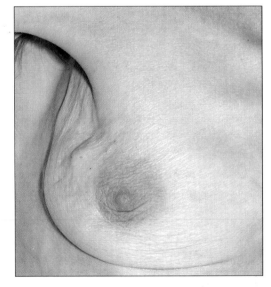

7.1 A breast mass. The cancer is rarely visible as a lump on inspection. This is more likely in the atrophic breast of the postmenopausal woman. The lump is clearly visible in the outer half of the right breast.

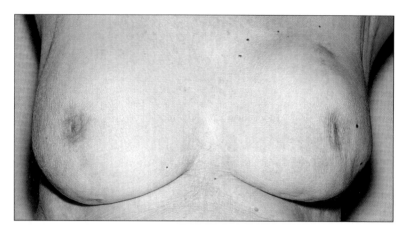

7.2 Lump and nipple retraction. This patient had a mass and nipple retraction on inspection of the left breast.

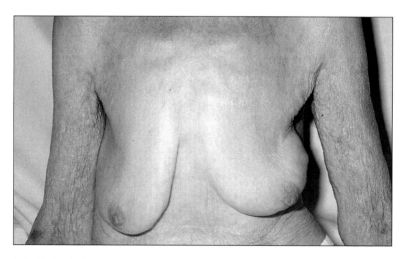

7.3 Altered nipple height. The breast cancer in the left breast has elevated that side so the nipple heights are different.

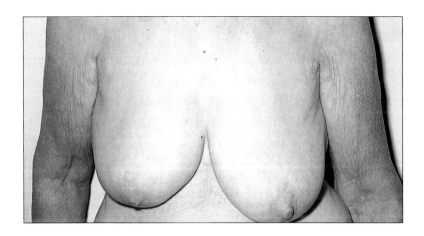

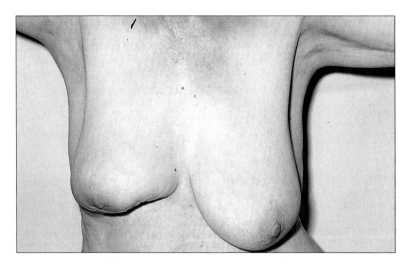

7.4 and 7.5 Inspection on arm elevation. It is a good practice to examine the patient sitting and with the arms elevated. This patient had no apparent abnormalities with her arms by her side (**7.4**, upper), but on raising her arms (**7.5**, lower) there was an obvious difference caused by the cancer in her right lower breast.

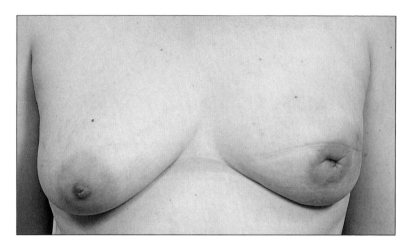

7.6 Nipple retraction. A subareolar cancer often produces nipple retraction, as in the left breast of this patient.

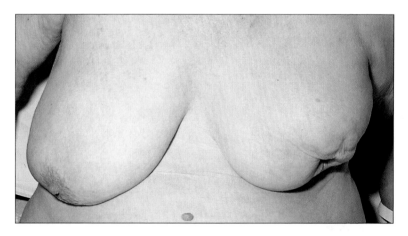

7.7 Breast distortion. Note the distortion and gross nipple retraction in the left breast. A schirrous carcinoma may give the appearance of a disappeared breast. This process may go on to erode the nipple, producing an 'automastectomy'.

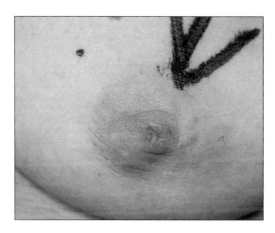

7.8 Areolar mass. This lesion causing a mass in the areolar skin at seven o'clock proved to be a slow growing tubular carcinoma of the breast.

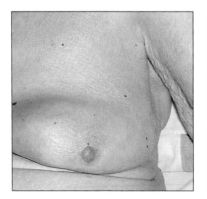 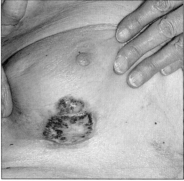

7.9 and 7.10 The hidden lesion. Cancers in the inframammary fold may be missed unless the pendulous breast (**7.9**, left) is elevated to inspect all the skin thoroughly. The cancer in this patient is easily demonstrated by simply lifting the breast (**7.10**, right).

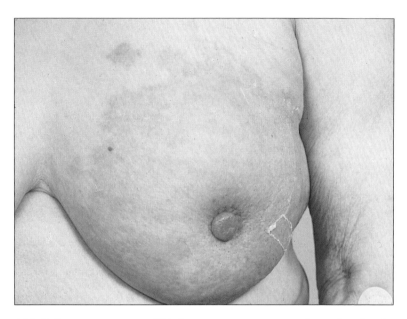

7.11 Inflammatory cancer. This is an uncommon aggressive variant involving widespread lymphatic involvement, leading to skin erythema and peau d'orange. The erythema is produced by an inflammatory response to the tumour and is not due to infection. This tumour is inoperable from the outset and requires chemotherapy as initial treatment. Note the nipple retraction and widespread erythema: this can occasionally be mistaken for an abscess if care is not taken in the examination.

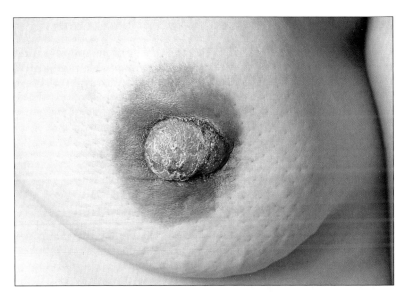

7.12 Peau d'orange. In this Asian woman, a large breast cancer is infiltrating the nipple with extensive peau d'orange, which is more marked in the lower half of the breast.

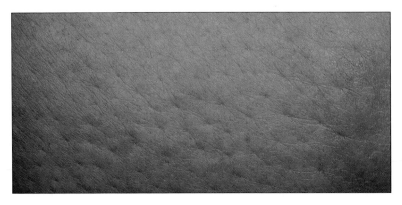

7.13 Peau d'orange: close-up. The orange peel appearance is produced by skin oedema emphasising the orifices of the skin sweat glands.

Mammographic Manifestations of Breast Cancer

With the widespread use of breast screening by mammography, many breast cancers are first diagnosed as impalpable radiological lesions. Commonly breast cancer is seen mammographically as a mass (spiculated or lobulated), architectural distortion of the breast, an area of microcalcification or an area of breast asymmetry.

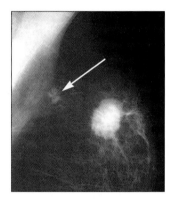

7.14 Breast cancer mammogram. This left breast mammogram shows a large well-defined carcinoma in the front of the breast with a second smaller carcinoma (arrow) close to the pectoral muscle posteriorly. It demonstrates the importance of mammography in palpable breast cancer as the second carcinoma was impalpable, but its presence indicated multifocality and the need for a mastectomy. Note the central spiculated opacity with irregular margins and a smaller opacity posteriorly.

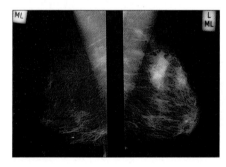

7.15 Large breast cancer mammogram. Mammograms may show large diffuse carcinomas. In the above example, a clear fatty upper half of the right breast is evident. In the left breast there is an asymmetric white density and a large diffuse carcinoma, which proved to be inoperable as it measured 10 cm in diameter.

7.16 Screen-detected breast cancer. This 1 cm cancer of the right breast was impalpable and can be seen (arrowed) lying close to pectoral muscle. Needle localisation biopsy showed it to be a tubular carcinoma. Microcalcifications are typical of ductal carcinoma *in situ* when present without an obvious mass lesion. They occur in 40% of breast cancers when they are usually associated with a mass.

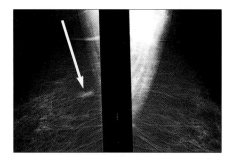

7.17 Specimen radiograph: needle localisation. Removal of impalpable mammographic abnormalities by a needle localisation technique requires radiography of the surgical specimen to confirm the lesion has been completely excised. This specimen radiograph shows an area of microcalcification associated with a small mass lesion adjacent to the end of the wire which turned out to be an invasive cancer. (See also Chapter 9, **9.19** and **9.20**.) Microcalcifications are typical of ductal carcinoma *in situ* when present without an obvious mas lesion. They also occur in 40% of invasive breast cancers when they are usually associated with a mass.

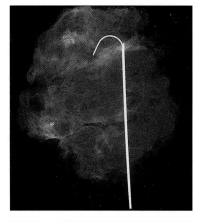

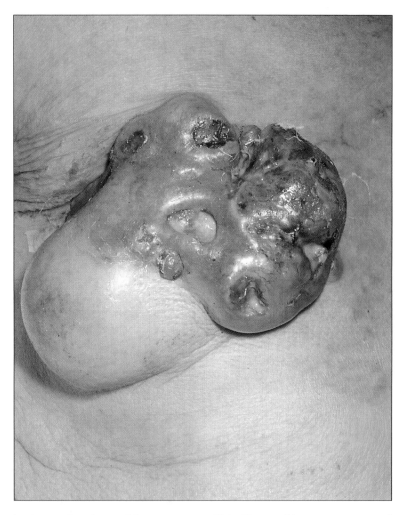

7.18 Locally advanced breast cancer. This 89-year-old woman presented with a protuberant mass replacing the upper half of her right breast. About 12% of breast cancer patients present with such advanced disease and it is an expression of denial as the patients actively conceal the obvious cancer.

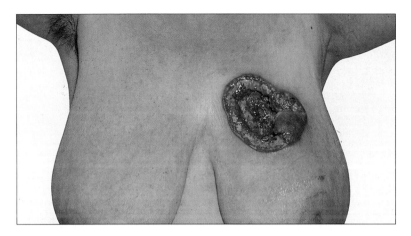

7.19 Ulcerating advanced breast cancer. This is a locally advanced T4 carcinoma of the left breast with an ulcerated base and a classical rolled edge. The deep infiltration of this tumour suggests that it is inoperable.

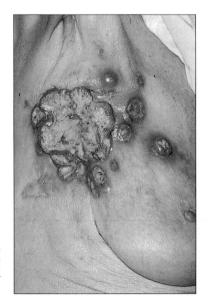

7.20 Satellite nodules. Carcinoma of the right axillary tail showing gross ulceration with satellite nodules.

91

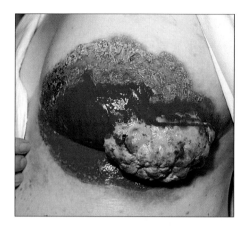

7.21 Bowenoid/Pagetoid spread. This locally advanced carcinoma shows ulceration in the lower half of the left breast with obvious intraepithelial cancer spread in the epidermis (Pagetoid spread), which is outlined by the large irregular red area at a distance from the main ulcer. Despite the extensive nature of the carcinoma there was no evidence of metastatic disease and wide resection with latissimus dorsi flap reconstruction was possible.

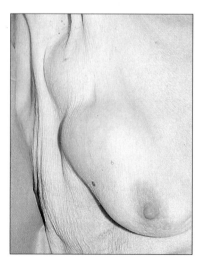

7.22 Lymphoma of the breast. This 89-year-old lady had undergone a tonsillectomy one year previously for a high-grade lymphoma. She presented with a mass in the upper outer quadrant of the right breast with an enlarged axillary node above. Biopsy confirmed a diagnosis of secondary lymphoma of the breast. Primary lymphoma of the breast is rare, but classically presents as a breast mass.

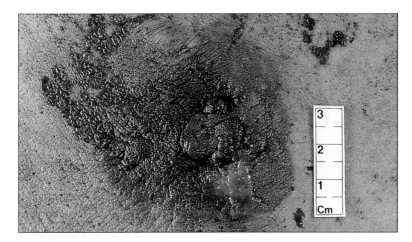

7.23 Primary angiosarcoma. The highly vascular appearance of this rare aggressive tumour is shown in this African patient. The histological appearance shows multiple vascular channels and the lesion is widely infiltrating and is resistant to both chemotherapy and radiotherapy. The 5-year survival is 10%.

7.24 Angiosarcoma after radiotherapy. This patient had undergone lumpectomy and radiotherapy for a left breast carcinoma some years previously and developed a rapidly growing brown purplish infiltration over most of the irradiated skin. Biopsy showed angiosarcoma, which was treated by wide excision and myocutaneous flap.

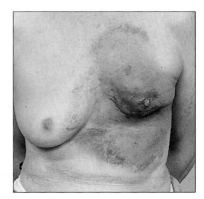

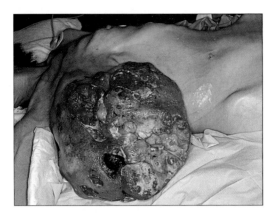

7.25 Fibrosarcoma. This patient actively hid the rapidly growing huge sarcoma of her right breast, which produced marked weight loss. The tumour came to light only when her landlady reported her to the general practitioner because of the foul smell. She underwent palliative resection, but died of lung metastases one year later.

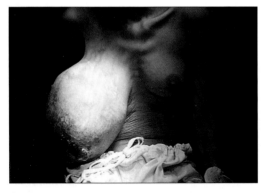

7.26 Rhabdomyosarcoma. An Indian patient with a rhabdomyosarcoma weighing 3 kg on excision arising from skeletal muscle of the right breast.

8 Breast Cancer: Recurrent and Metastatic

Since 70% of women who have their breast cancer treated will eventually develop either locoregional recurrence or metastatic disease it is important to recognise the pattern of recurrence at an early stage.

Recurrence may be local, regional (lymph nodes) or distant and usually occurs within the first five years of follow-up. Factors predisposing to local recurrence include: poorly differentiated tumours, lymphovascular invasion, and axillary node involvement.

Distant metastases from breast cancer occur predominantly in the skeleton, lungs and liver. Involvement of multiple sites is common. Bone metastases have a better prognosis than metastases to the liver or lungs and often respond to hormonal manipulation whereas faster growing liver metastases invariably require chemotherapy.

Bone metastases usually present with bone pain, although pathological fractures or hypercalcaemia also occur. Pain can be controlled by bisphosphonate therapy, analgesia, or irradiation of the lesion. Pathological fractures often require orthopaedic internal fixation and irradiation.

Lung involvement may declare itself by breathlessness or by the development of coin-shaped lesions on chest X-ray. Pleural effusions may require to be drained percutaneously.

Liver and brain metastases are life-threatening and need aggressive chemotherapy. Occasionally solitary brain metastases can be excised or irradiated to good effect.

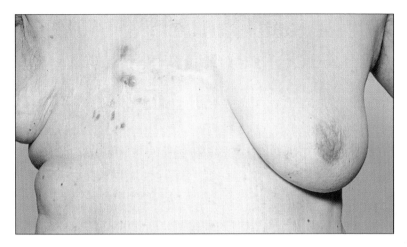

8.1 Local recurrence after mastectomy. Local recurrence may occur in the mastectomy flap wounds. It can be separated into three types: a single flap recurrence, which is best treated by wide excision followed by radiotherapy; raised red nodules (as in this picture); or diffuse infiltration.

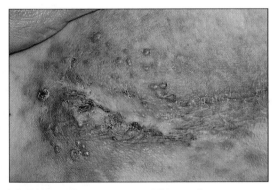

8.2 Diffuse flap recurrence. This carries a poor prognosis and is often the harbinger of, or appears simultaneously with, distant metastases. This patient developed multiple flap recurrence with visible raised nodules and associated with skin erythema. It is very difficult to treat such recurrence surgically.

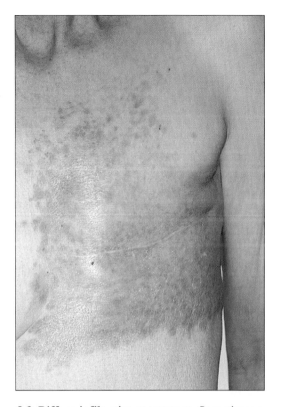

8.3 Diffuse infiltrative recurrence. Sometimes a diffuse infiltrative recurrence occurs throughout the skin of the mastectomy flaps. Tumour cells can be found in the skin if it is biopsied. This type of recurrence often remains confined within the radiotherapy field and manifests as diffuse erythema as in this case.

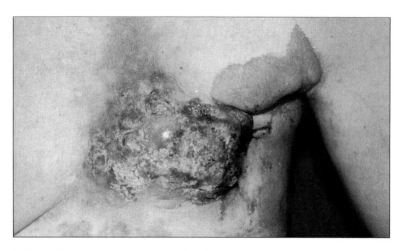

8.4 Local recurrence. More rarely local recurrence presents as an ulcerating mass, which often responds well to hormonal agents (e.g. tamoxifen or progestogen).

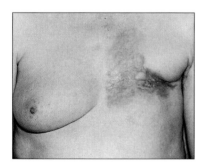

8.5 Local recurrence. Three months later the tumour is much smaller after teatment with tamoxifen.

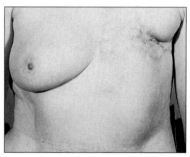

8.6 Local recurrence. By six months the disease has almost completely disappeared.

Local Recurrence after Conservation

Around 10–15% of women will develop breast recurrence after initial treatment of their primary breast cancer by wide local excision and radiotherapy. This frequency increases to 40% if radiotherapy is omitted. Breast recurrence can present clinically or radiologically.

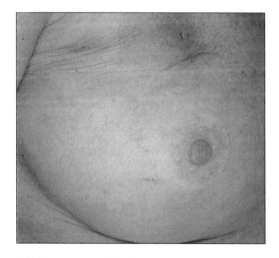

8.7 Recurrence after breast conservation treatment. This woman presented with a red lump in the medial end of her scar. As radiotherapy cannot be repeated, the woman requires a mastectomy to gain local control. An alternative is to carry out primary reconstruction of the breast after mastectomy using a myocutaneous flap.

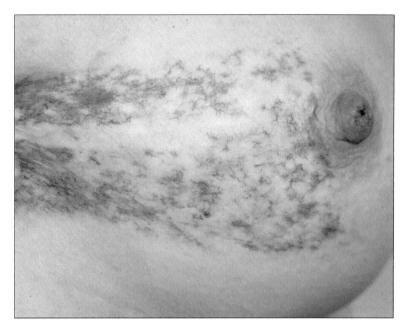

8.8 Occult recurrence. In this instance there is a bloody nipple discharge occurring two years after breast conservation. There was no palpable lump, but mammograms revealed an underlying mass lesion in the area of the scar and this patient required mastectomy. Note the cosmetically unattractive marked telangiectasia due to radiotherapy.

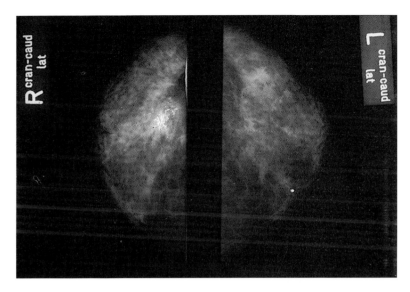

8.9 Mammogram of recurrence. Most women are followed up after breast conservation therapy by annual mammograms. The presence of a mass lesion or new microcalcification indicates the development of a recurrence or a new primary tumour. Note the microcalcification in the central area of the right mammogram behind the nipple. This was a second primary tumour associated with widespread ductal carcinoma *in situ*, which developed five years after breast conservation treatment.

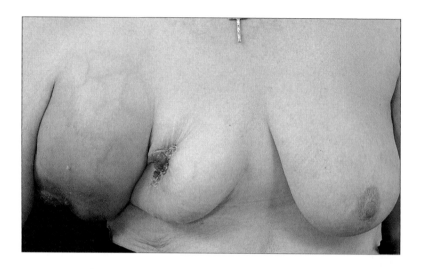

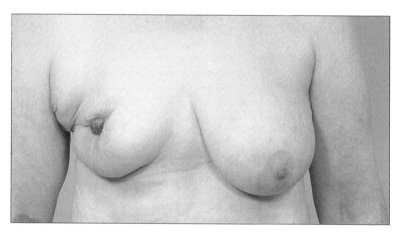

8.10 and 8.11 Axillary disease. Occasionally women present with a bulky axillary nodal mass associated with a smaller primary breast tumour. Note the large right axillary mass and ulceration of the breast above the nipple in the upper picture of this 60-year-old lady (**8.10**). Treatment with tamoxifen led to marked shrinkage of the axillary mass and breast disease (**8.11**, lower).

8.12 Axillary and breast recurrence. The frequency of axillary recurrence depends on the nature of the surgery and radiotherapy given to the axilla. Up to 30% of women with clinically negative nodes who have no surgery or radiotherapy to the axilla and 20% who have radical radiotherapy alone to the axilla develop axillary node recurrence compared with 5% treated by surgical axillary clearance. This Asian lady presented with a large palpable axillary mass and a mass in her breast underlying her wide local excision scar. Two years before she had wide local excision and was given tamoxifen for a small carcinoma of the breast. The scar recurrence was excised and an axillary node biopsied. Following this she was given radiotherapy to her breast and axilla.

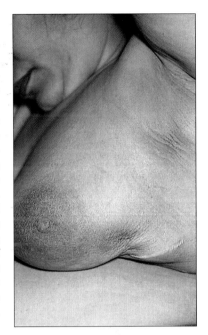

8.13 Ulcerating axillary recurrence. The axillary tumour ulcerated 11 months later and control was lost of both the axillary and breast disease. Bulky axillary disease is difficult to control by radiotherapy and is best dealt with by axillary clearance.

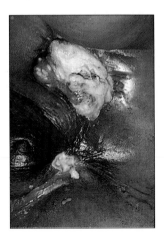

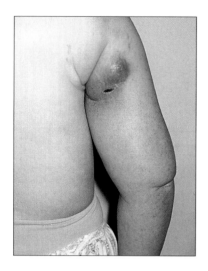

8.14 Axillary recurrence. This may lead to brachial plexus neuropathy by direct infiltration. Note the right axillary disease extending onto the posterior arm and associated with lymphoedema of the right arm, which is particularly marked above the elbow. It was associated with intractable excruciating pain along the ulnar nerve (medial) distribution of the hand.

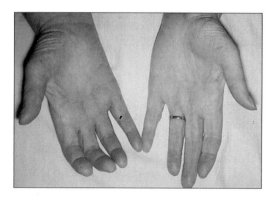

8.15 Hand signs of brachial neuropathy. The hands of the patient in **8.14** show wasting of the thenar and hypothenar eminences along with interossei (between the fingers) of the right hand. This occurs because of invasion of the T_1 motor and sensory nerve route leading to paresis. It is very difficult to treat and is best prevented by adequate initial surgery to the axilla.

Metastatic Disease

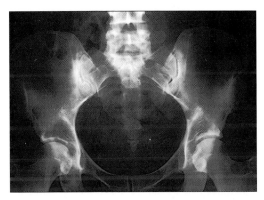

8.16 Bone metastases. These occur in up to 70% of women with breast cancer and commonly present with bone pain, pathological fracture, or hypercalcaemia. Note the multiple bony metastases in the pelvis of this woman, which manifest on a plain radiograph as radiolucent bones.

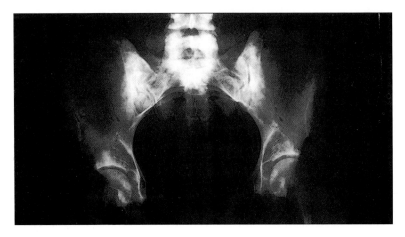

8.17 Bone metastases often respond to hormonal manipulation. They become more dense (sclerotic) as illustrated by this radiograph from the same woman as in **8.16** after treatment for six months with tamoxifen.

105

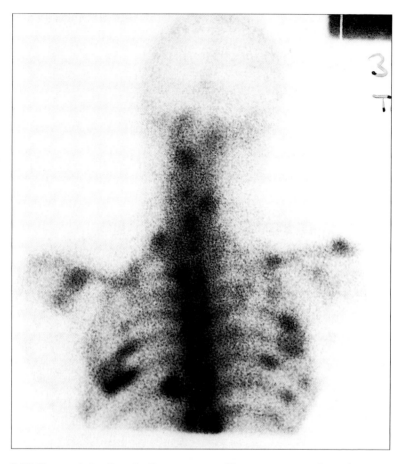

8.18 Bone pain is often the first symptom of bone metastases. It can however be confused with osteoporotic bone pain. A radioisotope bone scan is helpful and will often show multiple areas of uptake of isotope (dark areas on scan), which are called 'hotspots' of activity. The presence of such hotspots in the absence of any benign radiological lesion on plain radiograph of the area is indicative of bone metastases. Note the hotspots in the ribs and cervical spine.

8.19 and 8.20 Bone metastases on bone scan. Occasionally no lesions are visible on plain radiography and a repeat bone scan will be necessary to find out if there has been any response to hormonal manipulation. Note the diminished number of hotspots in **8.20** (lower) compared with **8.19** (upper). This indicates a response to therapy.

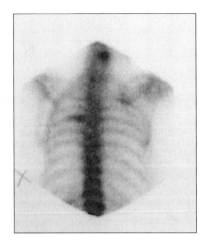

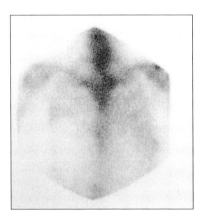

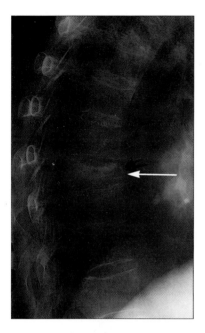

8.21 and 8.22 Pathological fractures.
These can occur in the long bones or
the spine. This lady had a collapsed
tenth thoracic spine vertebral body
due to a metastasis (**8.21**, upper,
arrowed). The bone scan shows a
corresponding hotspot in the
thoracic spine (**8.22**).

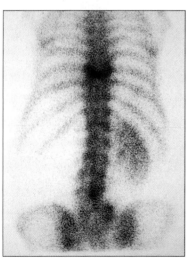

8.23 A more common fracture site in the neck of femur. In this case the orthopaedic surgeon will need to pin the femoral neck, and scrapings from the medullary cavity of the bone should be sent for histology to confirm the pathological nature of the lesion.

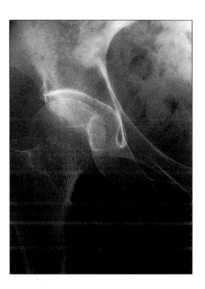

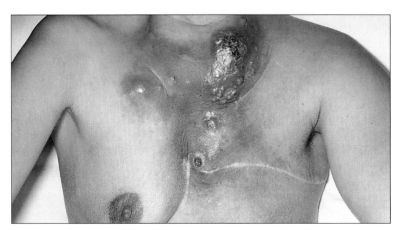

8.24 Recurrence in the mediastinal nodes. Recurrence in the mediastinal nodes that run alongside the internal mammary artery is rare. Radiotherapy does not always control such recurrence and they may ulcerate anteriorly between the costal cartilages. This lady also had large nodes around the root of the neck.

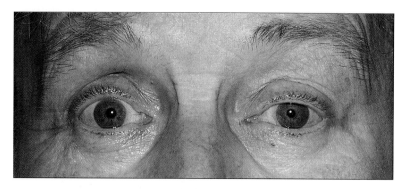

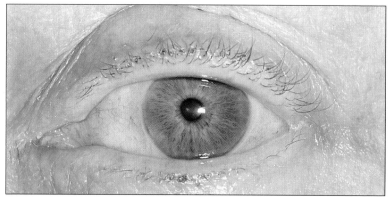

8.25 and 8.26 Recurrence in the mediastinal nodes. Alternatively mediastinal recurrence may declare itself by infiltration of the cervical symptomatic chain leading to Horner's syndrome. Note the ptosis of the left upper eyelid (**8.25**, upper) associated with a constricted left pupil (**8.26**, lower).

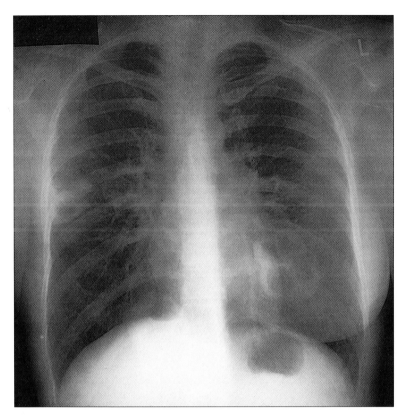

8.27 Pulmonary metastases. These manifest as shortness of breath or may be asymptomatic and noted on a coincidental chest radiograph. This chest radiograph shows several large masses in both lung fields with lucent centres. These represent large necrotic pulmonary metastases. Occasionally recurrence take the form of diffuse infiltrations of the lungs leading to progressive shortness of breath (so-called lymphangitis carcinomatosa).

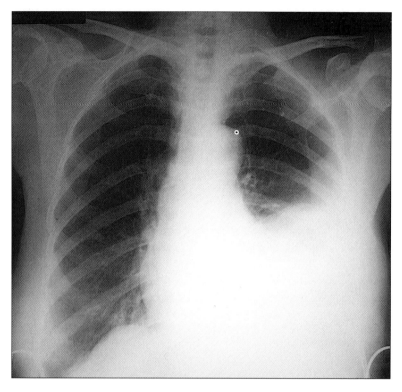

8.28 Pleural effusion. This patient presented with shortness of breath. She had undergone a left mastectomy for breast cancer in the past, and the chest X-ray shows a large left-sided pleural effusion.

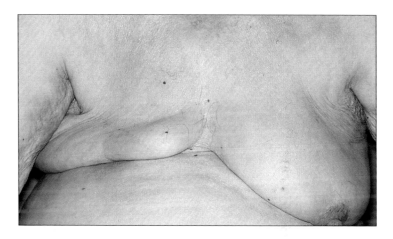

8.29 Liver metastases. The liver is the second most common site of metastasis from breast cancer and such metastases present with back pain, an enlarging liver, and progressive jaundice. Liver function tests usually have an hepatitic pattern with a raised transaminase. This patient presented with jaundice and an enlarged liver three years after her right mastectomy. Note the yellow skin and right mastectomy scar.

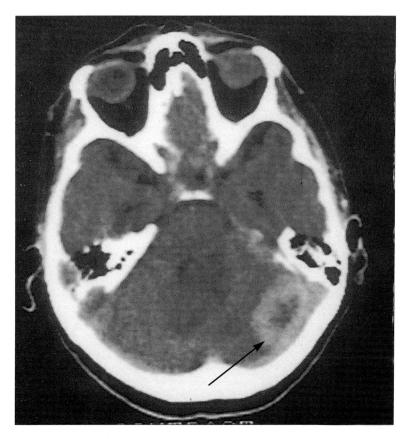

8.30 Brain metastases. This is a contrast-enhanced CT scan of the brain showing a cerebellar metastasis (arrowed) which is visible as a white ring with surrounding oedema.

9 Breast Cancer: Surgical Management

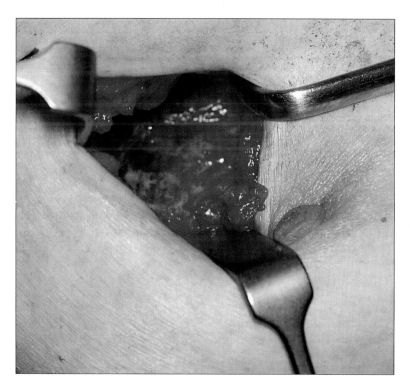

9.1 Breast biopsy. Despite the increasing use of needle aspiration cytology, and mammography, discrete lesions in the breast may remain a diagnostic problem and require removal by open biopsy. The essential principles are a cosmetically planned incision, good light, and adequate retraction as shown here. The smallest amount of tissue to produce a diagnosis should be removed with careful haemostasis. A subcuticular absorbable suture should be used to close the skin.

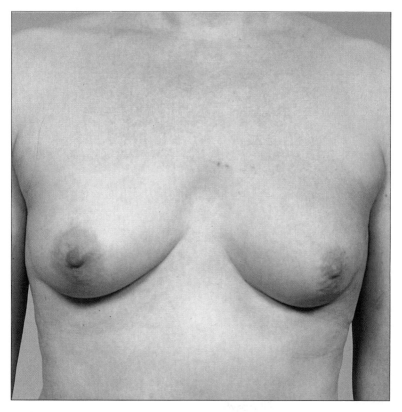

9.2 Wide local excision. A wide local excision can be performed with good results as shown here in a patient who had a small carcinoma removed from the left breast. The tumour and a minimum margin of 1 cm of breast tissue should be removed.

9.3 Wide local excision and axillary node clearance. Breast conservation should encompass a wide local excision and surgical clearance of the axillary nodes. Optimal cosmesis and minimal morbidity are obtained by using two separate incisions in Langer's lines of tension for the cancer excision and node clearance as shown here in the right breast.

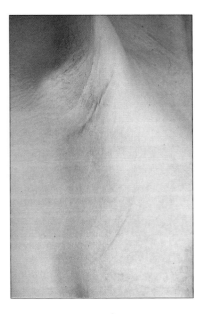

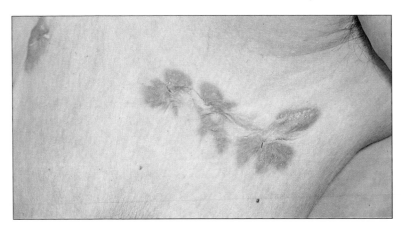

9.4 Keloid scar. Keloid scars may mar the final result and are unpredictable. The use of interrupted skin sutures here has resulted in a keloid scar at each skin puncture site.

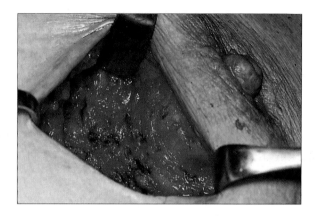

9.5 Quadrantectomy.. The photograph shows the operative appearance after quadrantectomy where a quarter of the breast has been removed up to and including the ducts entering the nipple base. The specimen is excised down to pectoralis fascia but only a small ellipse of skin is taken with the specimen. Quadrantectomy will usually leave some cosmetic deformity in the postoperative breast

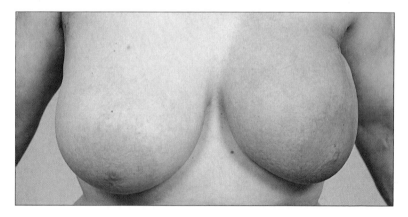

9.6 Post-breast conservation. An example of breast conservation by tumorectomy and radiotherapy showing the immediate post-radiotherapy erythema of the left breast.

118

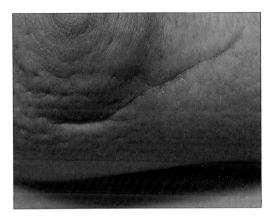

9.7 Post-radiotherapy. This shows localised oedema of the breast around the tumour excision scar after radiotherapy which is severe enough in this case to produce peau d'orange.

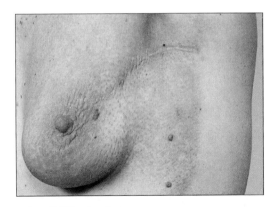

9.8 Post-breast conservation. *En bloc* resection by quadrantectomy of an upper outer quadrant cancer with axillary node clearance using one long excision often leads to oedema of the breast. Since radiotherapy must be given to the scar and tumour bed the radiation field may include the lower axilla as shown here. This results in elevation of the nipple with a poorer cosmetic result.

Conservation and Mastectomy Techniques

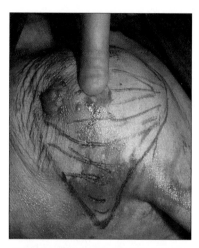

9.9 Making flaps for mastectomy. The finger points to a 5 cm carcinoma above the left nipple that had failed to respond to tamoxifen in an elderly woman. The flaps are marked with a 3 cm clearance around the tumour as shown.

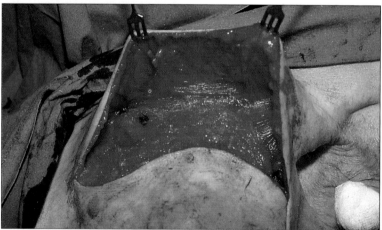

9.10 Dissection of the upper flaps up to the level of the clavicle. It is important to cut thin flaps to minimise recurrence.

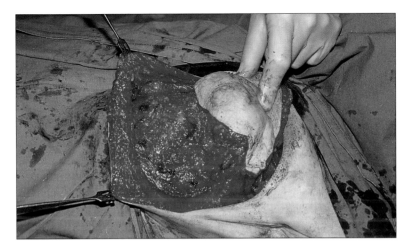

9.11 Lower and lateral flap dissection. Lower and lateral flaps dissected out inferiorly to the level of the rectus sheath and laterally to the edge of latissimus dorsi.

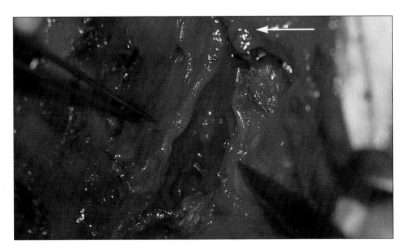

9.12 Completed axillary clearance. This shows the long thoracic nerve and thoracodorsal nerves (pointers) and the axillary vein above (arrowed).

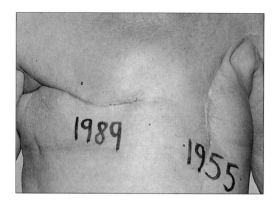

9.13 Changing fashions. A patient who had her first carcinoma in 1955 treated by left Halsted mastectomy and her second breast carcinoma treated by modified radical mastectomy (Patey) in 1989. Note the vertical scar on the left has now become oblique on the right and the loss of the pectoralis major muscle on the left, giving a poorer cosmetic result.

Complications of mastectomy

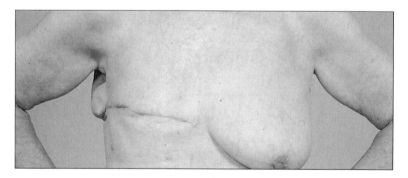

9.14 Complications of mastectomy. This patient has a 'dog ear' of skin in the right axilla after a mastectomy. Careful planning of the amount of skin excised is important in the elderly patient with lax skin.

9.15 'String sign'. A characteristic cord-like structure seen in the axilla or upper arm after axillary node clearance. This is often thought to be a thrombosed vein (as in Mondor's disease), but is in fact a fibrosed extension of the axillary suspensory ligament.

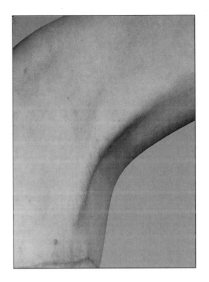

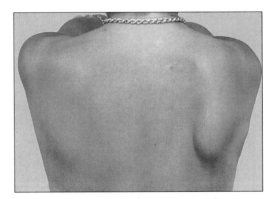

9.16 Winged scapula. This effect is due to the division of the long thoracic nerve, which supplies serratus muscle. As this muscle normally opposes the scapula to the rib cage, the loss of muscle power leads to winging of the scapula on flexion of the arm at the shoulder joint, seen on this patient's right side.

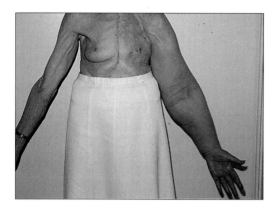

9.17 Lymphoedema. This patient has gross lymph-oedema of the left arm. Thirty years before she had radical mastectomy and radical radiotherapy to her axilla. There is an increased incidence of severe lymphoedema when both surgery and radio-therapy are given to the axilla.

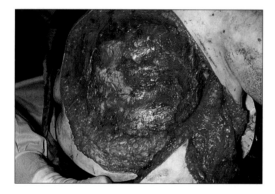

9.18 Radical mastectomy. The more extensive dissection used in Halsted's mastectomy is shown here after removal of the left breast and pectoral muscles, leaving the ribs and intercostal muscles on the chest wall.

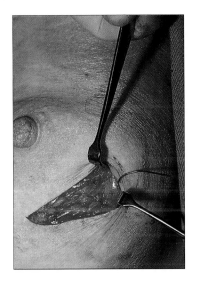
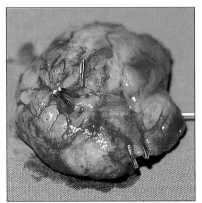

9.19 and 9.20 Needle localisation biopsy. The left-hand photograph (**9.19**) shows an operative approach to a mammographic abnormality which has been localized with a wire placed preoperatively. The incision is made close to the entrance of the wire into the skin, and the wire is followed down to the abnormal area which is then excised and sent for specimen radiography to confirm that the correct area has been removed. The right-hand photograph (**9.20**) shows the removed specimen with the wire entering from the right-hand side, with the end of the wire embedded in the specimen. Small metal clips are placed to mark the different margins of the removed tissue in order to allow the pathologist to identify each margin. This allows the location of any histologically involved margin to be determined so that further surgery can be planned with a view to removing the tissue adjacent to the involved margin.

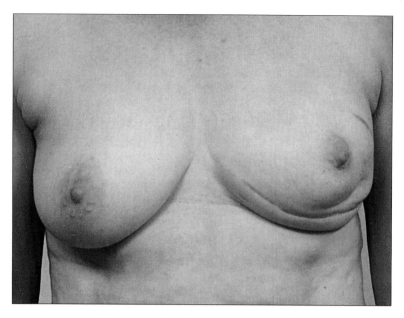

9.21 Subcutaneous mastectomy and reconstruction. This patient has undergone subcutaneous mastectomy for widespread ductal carcinoma *in situ* (DCIS) in her left breast. This operation does not always produce a good result because the lower one third of the breast overlies the serratus muscle and a simple subpectoral implant tends to be too high. The alternative subcutaneous implants have a high rate of fibrous capsular contraction and may extrude through the thin skin flaps. The nipple ducts may occasionally be a nidus for progress of a DCIS. This could be avoided or reduced by either nipple excision or irradiation of the nipple.

Breast Reconstruction Techniques

Breast reconstruction (**9.22–9.28**) after a mastectomy may be performed using tissue expanders, which avoid additional scarring but take longer than a simple implant or myocutaneous flap reconstruction because the skin expansion has to be carried out gradually.

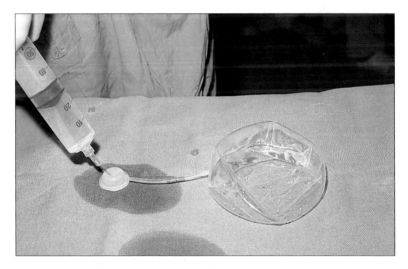

9.22 Tissue expander. The expander consists of a large expandable bag connected by a small tube to the port that has a silicone dome and metal backplate, which allows intermittent percutaneous puncture by a needle as shown. Saline or water is injected at 1–2 weekly intervals to stretch the skin of the chest wall gradually. On withdrawing the needle the silicone rubber dome of the port acts as a self-sealing valve.

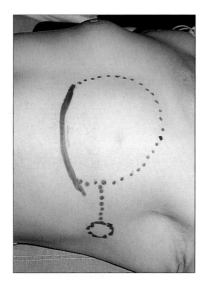

9.23 Positioning the expander bag. The skin marking on the left chest (the site of a previous left mastectomy) shows the intended position of the expander bag under the pectoralis major muscle. The dotted line and small circle in the axilla indicate the position of the filling tube and port.

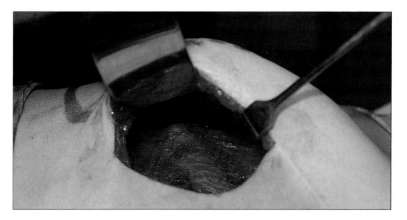

9.24 Inserting the expander. The subpectoral space beneath pectoralis major muscle has been opened up to insert the expander. The patient is in the same orientation as in **9.23**. Note the rib seen in the base of the pocket.

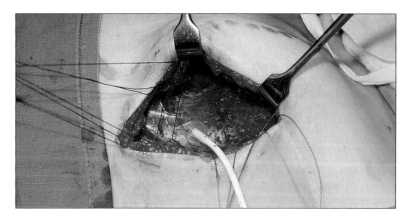

9.25 The expander bag is placed in the subpectoral pocket. The bag is empty at this stage, but will be partially filled at the end of the operation using the filling tube seen in the lower part of the picture.

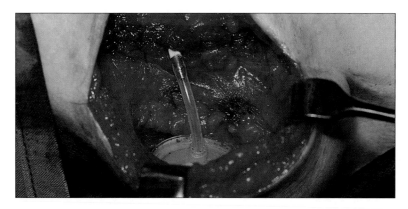

9.26 The secondary pocket for the port is made in the axilla. The port and tubing are connected up and placed in the pocket. The expander bag is now fully in the subpectoral pocket and the muscle has been closed around it leaving the filling tube coming from the pocket as shown in the upper part of this picture.

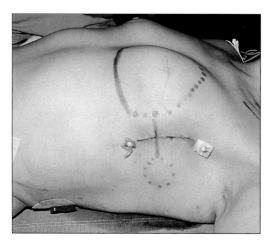

9.27 The final postoperative result with a small volume of fluid in the expander. Further filling and expansion will take place over the next 1–6 months to obtain full expansion.

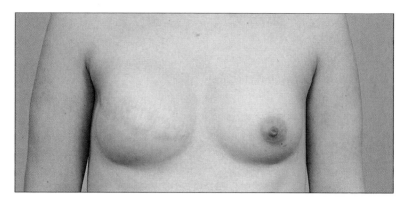

9.28 The final result in a different patient. This shows the completed reconstruction on the right side after replacing the expander with a silicone gel implant.

Breast reconstruction: latissimus dorsi myocutaneous flap

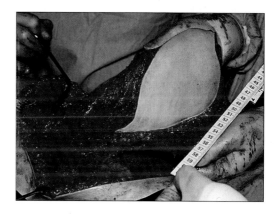

9.29 Latissimus dorsi myocutaneous flap: technique. The latissimus dorsi muscle is raised from the back with an 'island' of skin all from the back, which will form the new skin at the front of the reconstructed breast. The patient is lying on her side and her head lies to the left. A skin island measuring 20 cm long by 10 cm wide can be easily raised.

9.30 Latissimus dorsi myocutaneous flap: the completed reconstruction. This shows the skin island forming the new left breast skin and sutured to the upper and lower mastectomy flaps. The bulk of the breast is form- ed by an underlying silicone gel prosthesis because the latissimus dorsi muscle has insufficient bulk by itself to fill out the breast. Note the good colour match of the flap skin to the chest wall skin.

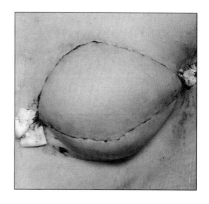

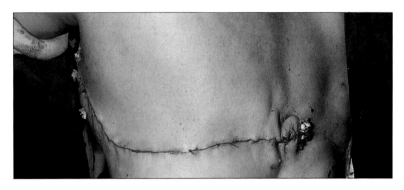

9.31 Latissimus dorsi myocutaneous flap: the horizontal back wound. This is produced by removing the skin island and transposing the latissimus dorsi flap. If it is kept horizontal it can be hidden by the back strap of the bra. The flap has been raised from the patient's left side and the patient's head is at the top.

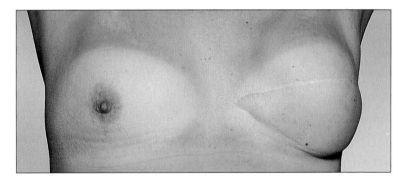

9.32 Latissimus dorsi myocutaneous flap: the final result. The completed left breast reconstruction (without a nipple) in a young woman. The skin island has a good colour match with the chest skin and the patient has good symmetry and volume. The distribution of the sun tan shows that this patient has gone back to wearing her bikini swimsuit and is a clear sign of the patient's confidence in her breast reconstruction.

Delayed breast reconstruction: rectus abdominis myocutaneous flap

This reconstruction (**9.33–9.38**) uses abdominal skin and fat, which is transposed to the chest wall on the rectus abdominis muscle and has the advantage that it usually has sufficient bulk to form the whole reconstruction without needing an implant.

9.33 Rectus abdominis myocutaneous flap. This shows the skin marking of the flap which is to be raised on the right rectus muscle and used to reconstruct the opposite (left) breast. The approximate course of the main vessel (superior epigastric artery) is shown in the upper half of the slide. Areas 1, 2 and 3 will be preserved, but area 4 (crosshatched) will be discarded because it is a long way from the muscle blood supply.

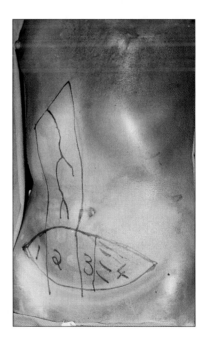

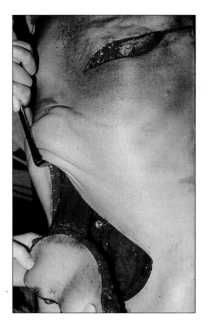

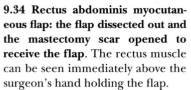

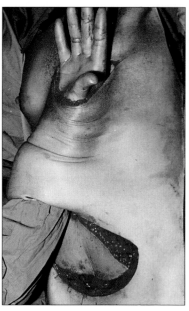

9.34 Rectus abdominis myocutaneous flap: the flap dissected out and the mastectomy scar opened to receive the flap. The rectus muscle can be seen immediately above the surgeon's hand holding the flap.

9.35 Rectus abdominis myocutaneous flap: the 'tunnel' between the abdomen and the chest wall. This is demonstrated by passing the surgeon's hand from the abdomen to the chest. The abdominal skin and fat in the flap will be similarly passed up to the chest wall once the rectus muscle has been freed up to the costal margin.

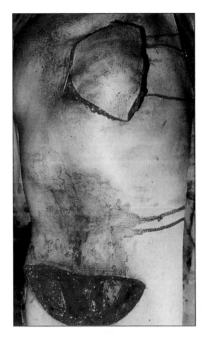

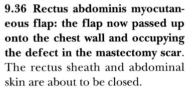

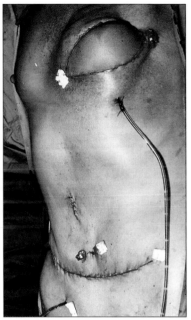

9.36 Rectus abdominis myocutaneous flap: the flap now passed up onto the chest wall and occupying the defect in the mastectomy scar. The rectus sheath and abdominal skin are about to be closed.

9.37 Rectus abdominis myocutaneous flap: the completed operation. This shows the closed abdominal flap tailored and sutured to the chest wall skin. Drains have been inserted to the chest wound and abdominal wound. The umbilicus has been repositioned because of the movement in the abdominal skin needed to close the abdominal wound.

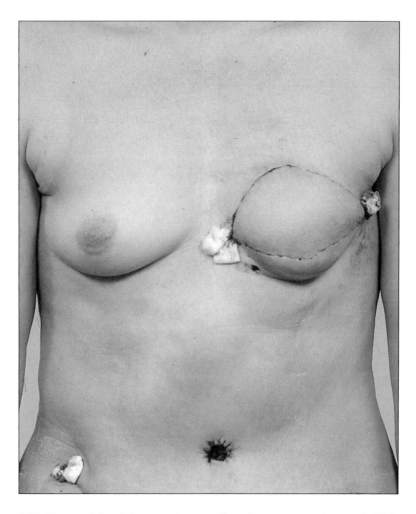

9.38 Rectus abdominis myocutaneous flap: the postoperative result. This shows a good skin match and volume and no implant is needed. An added advantage is the automatic abdominal lipectomy this operation produces and this procedure is currently much more popular with surgeons carrying out many breast reconstructions.

Nipple reconstruction

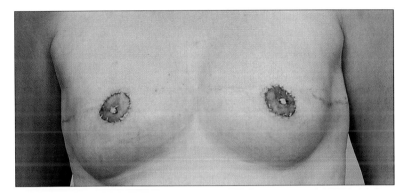

9.39 Bilateral nipple reconstruction after breast reconstruction by tissue expansion. The new 'nipples' have been formed from a local skin flap ('skate flap') and the areolar skin is mimicked by full thickness skin grafts taken from the inner thigh, giving a reasonable pigmented skin appearance. The skin darkening can also be produced by tattooing.

9.40 Nipple reconstruction using an areolar skin graft and an alternative nipple flap ('mushroom flap'). Close-up of an early postoperative result.

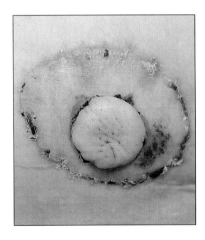

Complications of breast reconstruction

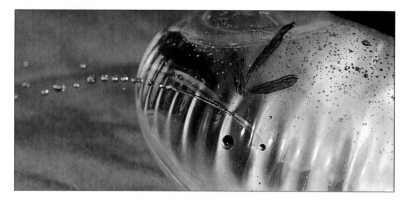

9.41 Ruptured saline prosthesis. This photograph shows the typical stress fracture (fold flaw) that affects a large number of saline-filled prostheses after some years of use. A small crack (shown by the red arrow) develops and the saline escapes, as shown.

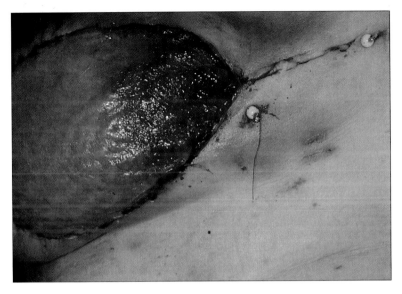

9.42 Flap necrosis. A left breast reconstruction using a latissimus dorsi flap which shows about a 30% necrosis of the flap extending from the axilla medially. Note the purple-black necrotic skin with surrounding erythema with a fairly marked demarcation line between the dead and living skin. The dead skin is the tip of an iceberg, as much larger areas of necrosis in the underlying fat and muscle will be present. Immediate excision of the dead tissue is required.

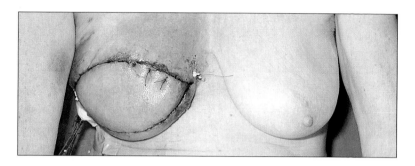

9.43 Infected implant. This patient developed an infection around the implant, which was put in as part of her latissimus dorsi flap reconstruction on the right side. Note the widespread erythema and oedema signifying a deep and extensive infection. In this situation the implant nearly always has to be removed, although it can be replaced later when the infection has settled.

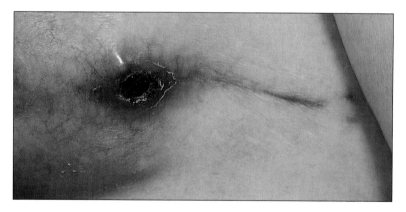

9.44 Extrusion of an implant. This patient developed an infection around her implant in the left side and the overlying scar broke down to reveal the shiny surface of the implant, which can be seen in the centre of the broken-down scar. As the implants are invariably infected or soon become so, the implant must be removed to allow healing before replacement at a later date.

Index